Copyright © 2021 All rights reserved.

The content contained within this book may not be reproduced, duplicated, or transmitted without direct written permission from the author or the publisher. Under no circumstances will any blame or legal responsibility be held against the publisher, or author, for any damages, reparation, or monetary loss due to the information contained within this book, either directly or indirectly.

Legal Notice: This book is copyright protected. It is only for personal use. You cannot amend, distribute, sell, use, quote or paraphrase any part, or the content within this book, without the consent of the author or publisher.

Disclaimer Notice: Please note the information contained within this document is for educational and entertainment purposes only. All effort has been executed to present accurate, up to date, reliable, complete information. No warranties of any kind are declared or implied. Readers acknowledge that the author is not engaged in the rendering of legal, financial, medical, or professional advice. The content within this book has been derived from various sources. Please consult a licensed professional before attempting any techniques outlined in this book. By reading this document, the reader agrees that under no circumstances is the author responsible for any losses, direct or indirect, that are incurred as a result of the use of the information contained within this document, including, but not limited to, errors, omissions, or inaccuracies.

CONTENTS

INTRODUCTION 9

SWITCHING TO 'REAL' FOOD 13

6-9 MONTHS OLD 17

FRUITS 17

    Apple puree 17

    Pear puree 17

    Baked bananas puree 17

    Blueberry puree 18

VEGETABLES 19

    Broccoli puree 19

    Yam puree 19

    Pumpkin puree 19

    Carrot puree 20

    Baked beet puree 20

    Cauliflower and celeriac puree 20

PORRIDGES 22

    Millet flour 22

    Rice or pearl barley flour 22

    Millet flour porridge 22

    Brown rice porridge 23

    Pearl barley porridge 23

9-12 MONTHS OLD 24

FRUITS 24

    Baked apples, pears and blueberry puree 24

    Fresh apricot puree 24

    Plum and blueberry puree 25

    Apple-dewberry puree 25

    Mango pure 25

    Baked apples with raisins 26

VEGETABLES 27

    Carrot-nectarine puree 27

    Zucchini-basil puree 27

    Pumpkin and apricot puree 27

    Special spinach-potato puree 28

    Vegetable broth 29

PORRIDGES 30

    Oatmeal with grapes 30

    Rice porridge with apples and fig 30

HABIT FORMATION 31

1-1.5 YEARS OLD 34

FRUITS 34

    Fruit yogurt 34

    Avocado-banana yogurt 34

    Banana- prune puree 34

    Tofu with fruit 35

    Mango and yogurt puree 35

    Cheese raisin dessert 36

    Rice with fruit 36

    Rice with peaches 37

VEGETABLES 38

    Cabbage surprise 38

    Tomatoes with carrots and basil 38

    Leek, potato and cottage cheese 39

    Avocado, carrot and cucumber 39

Zucchini with cheese 40
Red lentil and apple puree 40
Zucchini with tomatoes and pasta stars 41
Cauliflower with cheese 41
Risotto with pumpkin 42
Vichyssoise 43
Celery root and carrot soup 43
Potatoes with parsnip and rabbit meat 44
Green fruit salad 44
Dried apricot with papaya and pear 45
Ginger syrup 45
Quince marmalade 45
Swiss fruit muesli 46
Flakes breakfast 46
Home muesli 47

VEGETABLES **48**
Apple and vegetables and lentil puree 48
Lentil with vegetables 48
Green pea puree 49
Carrot and chickpea puree 49
Lentil and chicken puree 50
Sweet vegetable puree 50
Green fingers 51
White bean and veal puree 51
Vegetables with cheese sauce 52
Roasted garlic 52
Cauliflower, paprika and corn puree 53
Green bean and basil puree 53
Pistou sauce (fennel and apple sauce) 54

SOUP 55
Broccoli soup 55
Minestrone 55
Green peas soup 56
Pea and zucchini soup 57
Creamy chicken soup with celeriac and potato 57

GROATS 59
Fresh pear and semolina 59
Buckwheat and tofu 59
Buckwheat and vegetables 60
Couscous 61

EGGS AND COTTAGE CHEESE 62
Scrambled eggs 62
Eggs cooked in Bain Marie 62
Parmentier eggs 63
Carrot curd croquets 63
Curd croquets with cherry sauce 64
Fruit curd dessert with bread 65

BAKING 66
Pearl bread 66
French toasts 66
Raisin nut cookies 67
Strawberry rice pudding 68

FROM 3 TO 7 69
Taste of joy 69
Garden on your window sill 69
Home diplomacy 69
No TV! 70
Strict regime 70

Daycare 70

Approximate daily ration for 3-6 years old child 71

3-6 YEARS OLD 72

SALADS 72

Steamed vegetable salad 72

Fresh vegetable salad 72

Salad dressing 73

Chinese cucumber salad 73

Hawaiian salad with chicken 74

SOUPS 75

Pumpkin soup with orange 75

Carrot and lentils soup 75

Zucchini boats 76

Vegetable cutlets 77

Vegetable kebab 78

Ratatouille 78

Spanish omelet 79

Spaghetti with fish, raisins and pine nuts 80

Fish sticks 80

Chicken rolls 81

Veal with sweet potato 82

Rabbit with crostini 83

Small cutlets 83

Kebab on sticks 84

PASTRY AND DESSERTS 86

Pancakes for breakfast 86

Apricot puree 86

Muesli cookies 87

Carrot halva 87

Cream cheese bread 88
Curd rice pudding 89
Apple pie with raisin and hazelnut... 90
Curd roulade with candied fruits 91

AFTER 7 YEARS 93

BREAKFAST 93

Granola – homemade muesli 93
Omelette roll-ups 93
Omlette with secret.. 94
Filling with tomatoes 95
Filling with chicken and cucumber 95
Secret tomato sauce.. 95
Lavash and sweet pepper.. 96
Guacamole for children.. 97
Sweet bar "Health" 97
Meat casserole 98
Homemade hamburger with chicken cutlet 99
Banana cupcake 100

HOT MEAL..101

Spaghetti with chicken liver... 101
Spaghetti with sweet pepper 101
Potato with filling... 102
Potato pie with meat... 103
Meat and vegetables in a wok 104
Sole with grapes 105
Fish rissoles 105
Fish casserole 106
Turkey cutlets with beans 107
Spicy chicken 108

    Chicken with mushrooms 109

PASTRY, DESSERTS 110
    Curd rosettes 110
    Muffins with blueberry 110
    Curd croissants 111
    Chocolate cheesecake 112
    Poppy rolled cake 113
    Carrot cake with almonds 114

INTRODUCTION

I decided to write this book when I had my first child Marusya. I still can remember myself being 26 – my baby is crying in my arms because she has a stomachache. I love my husband very much, and before my daughter was born, he used to be the most important person in my life, but now there're two of them. And I'm so confused, because I don't know what to do: fry patties, express milk, do a belly massage or cook dill water. And there is no one to help, to give a piece of advice, because I'm far away from home and phone call is too expensive and no one has heard of Skype yet.

Well of course some people may say that you are a grownup if you are 26. I agree, but the thing is, it's easy to be a grownup, when you are surrounded by mommies-babysitters, grandmas, pediatricians and your friends, always ready to give some useful and practical advice. And when you're in another part of the world without any book, which says what to do and how to do…

Of course I had some books about pregnancy and children, when I was at home and haven't gone to America yet, but they were dull medical directory or just didn't have answers for my questions. I badly needed a book – a friend who can give me some smart and kind advice – a book in which I could read about experience of a mother like me, but who has already raised her children.

It's funny that when the baby is born, you think you'll remember it for the whole life. You think you won't forget how to express milk, how to cook puree or when to give dill water. Time passes by, your child now eats the same food as you, and there is no need to do a belly massage or pass vegetables and meat through a sieve. And I was sure that I knew everything well. No doubt! I've been through this! However, when another baby is born, it goes from the start, so I decided to write everything down.

I started writing in a notebook, then I started another one and in the end, I had a book shelf full of my notebooks. I tried to cook some meals from baby food recipe books and I found out that they were dull and tasteless, and my children didn't want to eat them.

So, I started improvising with the recipes I know, making them easier, cheaper and tastier. Suddenly many of my friends became mothers and I knew I had something to share, so here we are!

If you read this book and get a desire to have another baby, I'll be very happy!

You and your child

There is a tradition in America to celebrate the expected birth of a child. So the close friend of mine, Nina Foch, an amazing actress who is known for her roles in Stanley Kubrick's «Spartacus» and «An American in Paris», was the one who organized my baby shower. She invited her friends, who came with useful presents. One of them gave me a baby backpack, and said that she had used 5 different backpacks, but this one was the best. I found out she was right. I carried both of my children in it and then gave it to my friend. Another woman brought me the best express milk machine. And I was so touched by how thoroughly they chose those presents and how much attention they paid to me.

And during this party while we were sitting in an amazing Italian restaurant, drinking lemonade and enjoying the view of sycamores these wonderful women started to tell me about the meaning of life, that soon I would understand it and etc. I smiled and thought that we, Russians, didn't have such a problem as finding the meaning of life. We knew it and there was no need to talk about it. And only after the birth of my daughter I realized what these ladies were talking about and how wrong I was. And now I can tell you for sure that the meaning of my life is my children.

A boy or a girl

The majority of parents are concerned with the sex of their expected child. For example, someone wants to have a daughter, another – a son. Some women even try to control it by diets or some wild unreasonable beliefs. I had a friend who was eager to bear a boy so she ate only potatoes, mushrooms, bananas and dates. And what is more interesting she cut cabbage and nuts out of her diet, because she was sure they would decrease the chances to conceive a boy. That's all very nice but the only thing that really matters is your future relationships with a child.

Son is the only man who fully belongs to a woman. But you can't be sure that his love will be as big as yours. Whereas girls…. I'm pretty sure that there are some features in me which I definitely inherited from my mother. And I'm proud of them, but there are some… I wish I could change them. Girls look carefully on their mother: the way she talks, the way she treats her husband and etc. Mother is always a role model for a girl. Even on the subconscious level.

In the end the only thing that matters is the fact that you give a birth to a child and you are responsible for its happiness. Putting Exupery in other words – you're responsible, forever, for what you have born.

Normal delivery vs. C-section delivery

I often think of Nina Foch because she has saved me from C-section delivery, which is usually made when emergencies occur. However, my doctor tried to convince me that it would be easy to regain figure after it. And my friend said 'Nonsense! You'll turn into an invalid person for 2 month. It's a serious surgical procedure, during which you'll be cut and only God knows how long you will spend in the hospital. And if you do it by yourself, you'll be fine very soon.'

And she was right. I had 'normal' delivery twice and could stand and go home almost the next day after it. By the way, I know how desperately you want to come back home, but be patient. It's better to stay for a day or two in the hospital. Just to make sure everything is under control.

Your beloved man

As for me the biggest stress for maternal instinct is to give your newborn baby to nurses, even for a minute. But lying-in is very hard for a woman and her body, and after that the only thing she wants is to sleep and relax. But she can't – she has to feed and swaddle her baby. I was very lucky, because my husband helped me a lot.

It is very important for a father and a child to be on the same page. For example, my husband, Andrew, was a coach and he taught Marusya and Petia how to swim. But he was so awkward at first! His child was 5 years old and he had to bathe him. He was afraid to «break this little creature» but when he finally started the child began to swim in the bathe! Can you imagine it? It was the happiest moment for my husband.

Breastfeeding: expectations vs. reality

Breastfeeding is necessary for raising a healthy child. Usually inexperienced mums, seeing the great amount of powdered baby milk, give up on breastfeeding. But it's a big mistake.

Maternal milk is a unique product. It contains probiotics, which protect a baby from various illnesses. Doctors say that breastfeeding not only makes your child healthier but also smarter. Yes, it is hard and sometimes painful but you shouldn't refuse to do it because of you fear.

As for me, there are only two reasons for breastfeeding refusal: diseases making it impossible to breastfeed and the necessity to take medicines incompatible with breastfeeding.

Don't ignore the fact that you should prepare yourself for breastfeeding during pregnancy. Some experts recommend washing your nipples with cold water and rubbing your chest with a rough towel. Or it is possible to underlay you bra with little pieces of rough fabric. Also you should let your breast breath sometimes (15 minutes in a day is enough). Repeat these procedures day after day and it will prepare your nipples for breastfeeding.

But be careful! If there is a threatened miscarriage such procedures can lead to premature birth. It this case, doctors recommend preparing your nipples by lanoline creams.

To be honest, there are a lot of problems during the breastfeeding: no milk, too much milk… You don't know what to do. But there is no need to panic or to get upset. If you have too much milk (I had this problem) you can always pump it out, by yourself or by using breast pumps. As soon as you realize that there are no any disasters with breastfeeding – only small problems or inconveniences – you will relax and understand that the devil is not as black as it is painted.

The diet for mums

The most important thing during pregnancy is to eat healthy. There is a lot of information about diets for future mothers, but, please, be careful. To eat healthy doesn't mean to restrict yourself and do a lot of exercises. You can eat whenever you want but only healthy food. Some ladies are sure that during pregnancy they can eat white bread with butter and it will increase the amount of milk in the future. But the only thing that it will increase is your bottom. Sorry, ladies.

You should eat something that contains complex carbohydrate. For example, rice, spaghetti, couscous, sweet potato or just potato.

Doctors recommend eating bread, but don't go easy on it. If you want it so badly that can't resist, eat at least multi-grain bread. And don't forget about fruits and vegetables! You must eat them every day! Yes, some people are afraid of allergy, but it's nothing but a myth. The products you should avoid are veal, beef, farmer or cottage cheese and cheese. Try to replace them with products made from goat milk or pork, rabbit, turkey and porridges.

SWITCHING TO 'REAL' FOOD

I heard about a young couple, who after the birth of the baby, decided to go to the country to become farther from the city life and closer to nature. They grew their own vegetables and bought a cow. Everything seems to be fine; however, the parents thought that their child could tell them about the things he wanted or needed.

The thing that surprised me the most was that the parents didn't even realize that their six-month baby couldn't tell them to give him some grated squash or carrot. So when the mother ran out of breast milk, instead of starting giving vegetables they replaced breast milk with the cow one.

After three years they decided to come back to the city. 'Healthy life' has turned the child into a weak and thin boy with very pale skin. Doctors didn't know what to do, because the child refused to eat anything but milk.

I don't know how this story ends, but my point is that a six-month baby is fragile and helpless, and everything that concerns his feeding (when to eat and what to eat), depends only on you.

No need to hurry

I've read plenty of books about when it is better to start complementary feeding and I've come to a conclusion that it's better late than early because of the allergy and our current ecological situation. Women, who haven't fed their babies with breast milk, should be two times more careful when adding fruits and vegetables into the babies' diet, because their immune system is significantly different from those, who've consumed breast milk.

Doctors insist on milk being not enough for six-month babies. However, there are no strict rules when to start complementary feeding. World Health Organization advises to do it from six month, and according to our doctors you can start from four month. The best way to find out is to make a finger-prick blood test. If hemoglobin is below normal, then it's the right time for complementary feeding.

Getting to know the spoon

It's very important to start complementary feeding slowly (1/2 teaspoon is enough for the first time) and it's better to do it in the daytime. It will help you to find out if there is an allergic reaction or a diarrhea, which is difficult to notice at night. Don't worry if you hear belly rumbling, it's an ordinary reaction to the new food. In this case give some dill water. You can buy it or make by yourself: pour dill seeds in a glass, add boiling water and leave for 5 minutes, then drain through a few layers of gauze. If you notice any other allergic reactions such as rash or peeling, exclude this fruit or vegetable puree from the menu and stop complementary feeding for a week or two.

Feed the baby with breast milk at first, and then give some puree, because if the baby is hungry, he won't be impressed with your 'interesting' proposal.

Make sure puree you want to give is liquid, but don't pour it in a bottle! It's very important to teach your baby to chew. Use a plastic drinking bottle, which has 2-3 holes and comfortable handles. In fact the best way to give some new food is to give it on a finger. Yes! I'm not kidding! Wash your hands thoroughly and put a small amount of puree on your finger, and after some time you can give your baby a spoon. By the way, don't be afraid of a mess; teach him to eat by himself. Lay the floor with newspapers, put an apron on your little hero and give him a spoon. When the baby gets bored, feed him with a different spoon.

Wash or sterilize?

When the baby is born, you suddenly recognize that there are a lot of problems to solve, and the vital question is: what to do with teats and bottles? Is it better to sterilize them or just pour boiling water over them?

Don't go to extremes. Yes, it's compulsory to sterilize bottles, when the baby is younger than a year, but there is no sense in it after a year. When you kill harmful bacteria, you also kill beneficial ones. By the way, forget about antibacterial soap for the same reason. Babies have their own beneficial bacteria and if you get rid of them, who will protect your baby? A doctor from a TV advertisement?

Don't get me wrong, what I'm trying to say is – use common sense. My children swim like a fish. When Marusya was 8 month, I took her to the swimming pool. Many people said I went crazy, because it was a community pool, and I came with a small baby, but you can't disinfect everything around your child! Let him meet some bacteria, which live around. It doesn't mean you can dive or go to water parks, full of people. If you know that it's a small sport pool, where water is cleaned well, why not?

To cook or to buy

I've noticed that when mothers realize it's time to start complementary feeding, everyone runs to the nearest shop to buy some baby formulas, because they are easy to use. And you know that you can put them in your bag and feed your baby at any time.

I believe those baby formulas exist exactly for such cases, when you are in the road going somewhere, but if you are at home and you have energy for cooking, don't feed your baby with canned food.

I understand that we have to cope with fast rhythm of life, and most mothers work and sometimes don't have time for cooking. But there is a way out. At the weekend cook more than one portion of soup or puree and froze part of it in plastic containers. Don't leave them in a freezer for more than a month. It's better to heat the food using water bath or a special bottle warmer.

Check food's temperature. Put a few drops on the back side of you hand, if it doesn't hurt, the temperature is alright.

Don't give your baby the spoon you've used. Adults have too many bacteria, and sometimes we don't even know that we are ill. That's why I advise you to use different spoons.

Sugar alarm

Recent researches have showed that work of the baby receptors significantly differs from ours. What seems to be sweet enough for us is too sweet for the babies. That's why I don't recommend adding any sugar. And if you buy baby juice, it's necessary to dilute it with water. Otherwise you risk making your child addicted to sugar.

Porridges

Some doctors recommend starting complementary feeding with rice, because it doesn't contain gluten, so doesn't cause any allergies. Others believe the best porridge to start with is corn one.

You can buy baby rice cereals and add some breast milk or milk mixture to it, or rinse white rice with water, cook longer than usually, until very-very soft, pass through a sieve and blend in a blender. Don't add any salt or sugar, only some breast milk.

When your child is 6 month already, add corn and buckwheat porridges into his menu. After 7 month it's time to feed your child with oatmeal, millet or barley porridges. Cook semolina porridge only after a year.

Cultured milk foods

Everyone knows the value of cultured milk foods. But don't go easy on it. The big amount of, for example, kefir can affect the iron status and Hb level. It would be better to start drinking it since a child 8-9 months old.

Yolk and white

After 7 month you can try to eat yolks. If you have an allergy (and by "you" I mean your child) it's better to try quail eggs. And also you can start doing meat puree. I started with rabbit, because it is non-sensitizing. But it is possible to use veal or turkey. But avoid chicken as long as you can.

After a year the child can eat fish puree, but if you notice any allergic reactions, fish can wait for another year.

What to drink

The best variant is clear water. Definitely not from the tap – you need to filter and boil it for decontamination. But after these procedures the water becomes "dead". However, you can buy special water for children or you can do it at home. Pour filtered water into a bottle and let sit in the sun until chlorine residue disappeared. Then boil the water and put into the freezer. After freezing let it melt, but there should be an ice core. Also you can put a silver spoon in it. The water will be purified and decontaminated.

Allergy

I'm really lucky because my children don't have allergies. But I know that you need to work hard to understand it. You have to examine your child every day to understand on what products he has an allergic reaction. There is a list of the most common allergens: honey, nuts, eggs, milk, citrus cultures and etc. They are the first to be excluded from your children's diet.

My friend, Rita, has a son and he was highly allergic. She couldn't breastfeed him because of his reaction. She replaced breast milk with soymilk, but it didn't help. She spent so much money and time on hospitals, expensive clinics, medicines, but there was no result.

Once she had an appointment with a doctor in some small district hospital. The doctor appeared to be a wise and kind woman. She looked at Rita and her son and sighed: "Stop destroying the health of the boy by all these medicines. He needs a strict diet". She looked into patient's chart and gave Rita the list of allowed products: soaked in water for 8 hours potato, rabbit, buckwheat porridge, peeled green apple, whole-wheat bread and homemade kefir. Rita was shocked and the only question she could ask was: "And nothing else?" The doctor looked at her with a weary smile and said: "My dear, I've just had a patient who could eat only a boiled cabbage".

Without any other questions Rita put her son on this strict diet, and gradually they overcame their problem.

6-9 MONTHS OLD
FRUITS

Apple puree

It's better to use two sorts of apples: with sour and sweet tastes.

Ingredients:
- 2 cups apple, peeled and cubed;
- 1 cup water;

Process:
- Pour water in a medium saucepan, add apples and bring to a boil.
- Reduce the heat to low and cook for 12-15 minutes until tender, skimming off the scum if it appears.
- Blend until smooth, pass through a plastic sieve and cool.

Pear puree

Pears are very healthful because they create hostile environment for unfriendly bacteria.

Ingredients:
- 3 pears;
- 1 cup water;

Process:
- Wash the pears thoroughly, peel and finely chop.
- Pour water in a medium saucepan, add pears and bring to a boil.
- Reduce the heat to low and cook for 12-15 minutes.
- Blend until smooth.

Baked bananas puree

Ingredients:
- 2 bananas (do not peel);
- ½ cup water;

Process:

- Preheat your oven to 250F.
- Wash the bananas. On a waxed paper put the bananas and bake for 30 minutes.
- Put the bananas on a plate, peel them and cool for another 10 minutes.
- Place the bananas in a pot, add water and bring to a boil. Then place the mixture in a blender and blend until smooth and cool.

Blueberry puree

Ingredients:
- 2 cups blueberry;
- 1 ½ cup water;

Process:
- Pour water in a pot, add blueberry, bring to a boil, then reduce the heat and boil for another 10 minutes.
- Place the mixture in a blender and blend until smooth.

VEGETABLES

Broccoli puree

After broccoli is ready, use the broccoli broth to cook a soup for the whole family. Just add pasta, grated cheese and season with cream.

Ingredients:
- 2 cups broccoli florets;
- 4-5 cups water;

Process:
- Bring water to a boil, add broccoli, cover and cook until tender.
- Blend the florets until smooth. Add some broccoli broth if necessary.

Yam puree

For elder kids you can add 1 spoon of butter and a little pinch of sea salt and freshly ground pepper to the puree. It's a good side dish for chicken or meat patties.

Ingredients:
- 2 yams;
- 1 cup water;

Process:
- Preheat oven to 185 F.
- Wash the yams thoroughly, wrap with foil and bake for an hour until tender.
- Cool, peel and cut into cubes.
- Pour water in a saucepan, bring to a boil, add yams, bring to a boil again and turn off the heat.
- Cool and blend until smooth.

Pumpkin puree

Pumpkin is one of the most delicious vegetables, besides there are a lot of nutrients in it: protein, carbs, fat, sugars, and etc.

Ingredients:
- 1 lb pumpkin;

- 2 ½ cup water;

Process:
- Peel the pumpkin, cut it into cubes. Put in a pot, add some water, and bring to a boil. Reduce the heat and boil for another 25 minutes until tender. Cool on another pot
- Pour the broth into a blender and blend until smooth. Add some water if needed.

Carrot puree

Ingredients:
- 1 ½ cup carrots (cut into small cubes);
- 1 cup water;

Process:
- Put the carrots in a pot, add some water, bring to a boil, reduce the heat and boil until tender.
- Drain boiled water in another dish. Place the carrots in a blender and blend until smooth. Add the broth if needed.

Baked beet puree

For elder kids you can cook a simple salad. Just mix lettuce, goat cheese, little olive oil, few drops of apple vinegar and your favorite nuts.

Ingredients:
- 3 big beets;
- 1 cup water;

Process:
- Wash the beets thoroughly, wrap with foil and bake for about 40 minutes, until tender.
- Cool, peel and cut into cubes.
- Pour water in a saucepan, bring to a boil, add beets, bring to a boil again and turn off the heat.
- Cool and blend until smooth.

Cauliflower and celeriac puree

It can be a great garnish to fish instead of mashed potatoes! Adults also appreciate it especially if you add some olive oil, and sprinkle it with garlic and lemon juice.

Ingredients:

- 2 cup cauliflower;
- ½ cup celeriac (cut into cubes);

Process:

- Put the cauliflower and celeriac in a pot, add some water, and boil until ready.
- Drain water in another dish.
- Place the vegetables in a blender and blend until smooth. Add the broth if needed.

PORRIDGES

Now you can find a variety of cereals in shops: wheat, barley, rice, which are very useful if you want to cook porridge fast. But if you can't to find these cereals, you can make flour from grains at home. Keep the made flour in a plastic container in the fridge.

For elder children you can add a teaspoon of honey, maple syrup or homemade jam, especially if it was made without sugar (e.g., fruits and berries cooked in apple juice).

Millet flour

Ingredients:
- 1 lb millet;

Process:
- Preheat oven to 175 F.
- Rinse in water.
- Pour the millet in a baking sheet for an hour.
- Rinse in water again and put back in the oven to prevent bitter taste.
- Grind in a coffee grinder.

Rice or pearl barley flour

Ingredients:
- 1lb grains;

Process:
- Rinse in water.
- Fry in a dry pan for 3-5 minutes, stirring constantly.
- Cool and grind in a coffee grinder.

Millet flour porridge

Ingredients:
- 2 cup millet flour;
- 5 cup boiled water;

Process:

- Pour the water in a bowl and mix the millet flour without any lumps.
- Boil for 10 minutes on a low heat.
- Add some butter to taste.

Brown rice porridge

Ingredients:
- 2 cup brown rice flour;
- 5 cup hot boiled water;

Process:
- Pour the water in a bowl and mix the brown rice flour without any lumps.
- Boil for 10 minutes on a low heat.
- Cool for 45 minutes before serving.

Pearl barley porridge

Ingredients:
- 2 cup pearl barley flour;
- 5 cup hot boiled water;

Process:
- Pour the water in a bowl and mix the pearl barley flour without any lumps.
- Boil for 20-30 minutes on a low heat.

9-12 MONTHS OLD
FRUITS

Baked apples, pears and blueberry puree

If you combine this puree with yogurt, you will get a healthful breakfast for the whole family.

Ingredients:

- 3 apples;
- 3 pears;
- ½ cup blueberry;
- 1 cup water

Process:

- Preheat oven to 355 F.
- Wash the apples thoroughly, core them, but don't peel.
- Bake for 30-40 minutes.
- Peel the baked apples.
- Peel and cut pears, then put them in a saucepan.
- Add blueberry and water and bring to a boil. Simmer for 10 minutes over low heat.
- Mix apple, pears and blueberry and blend until smooth.

Fresh apricot puree

It's better to make apricot puree with fresh apricots. Do not feed your baby with apricots from grocery.

Ingredients:

- ½ lb apricots;
- ½ cup water;

Process:

- Pour water in a pot, add pitted apricots, bring to a boil, reduce the heat and boil for another 15 minutes.
- Place the mixture in a blender and blend until smooth.

Plum and blueberry puree

Ingredients:
- 3 stoned plums;
- 1 cup blueberry;
- ½ cup water;

Process:
- Pour water in a pot, add pitted plums and blueberry, bring to a boil, reduce the heat and boil for another 5 minutes.
- Place the mixture in a blender and blend until smooth. Add some water if needed.

Apple-dewberry puree

If you use sweet apples, you don't need any sugar.

Ingredients:
- 2 apples;
- 0,45 lb dewberry;
- 2 tbsps water

Process:
- Peel, core and cube the apples.
- Add all the ingredients in a small saucepan and stew for 15-20 minutes, until apples are tender.
- Blend until smooth and pass through a sieve.

Mango pure

Make sure your child isn't allergic to mango. Use only ripe mangoes, without dark spots and fiber.

Ingredients:
- 1 mango;
- 1 cup water;

Process:
- Wash the mango thoroughly, peel and cube.
- Add mango and water in a small saucepan, bring to a boil and cook for 5 minutes over low heat.

Baked apples with raisins

Drop the last point for older children.

Ingredients:

- 2 apples;
- 1/2 cup apple juice of water;
- 2 tbsps raisins;
- 1 tsp honey or maple syrup;
- 2 tsp butter;
- 2 little pinches cinnamon;

Process:

- Preheat oven to 355 F.
- Wash apples thoroughly, core and pierce with a fork.
- Put apples in the baking dish and pour juice or water around them.
- Stuff apples with raisins, add cinnamon, cover with honey of syrup if apples aren't sweet and grease the top with butter.
- Pour water in a saucepan, bring to a boil, add yams, bring to a boil again and turn off the heat.
- Bake for 45 minutes.
- Peel the apples and blend them until smooth. Add some water from the dish if necessary.

VEGETABLES

Carrot-nectarine puree

If you add yogurt, few drops of vanilla extract and a teaspoon of honey to this puree, you will get a tasty breakfast for the whole family.

Ingredients:
- 3 nectarines;
- 1 cup carrot, peeled and cut into small cubes;
- 1 cup water;

Process:
- Wash nectarines thoroughly, remove the pits and cut.
- Pour water in a saucepan and add nectarines and carrots. Bring to a boil, reduce the heat and cook for 20 minutes until tender.
- Cool and blend until smooth.

Zucchini-basil puree

Basil has a very strong taste, so for the first time use only one leaf, and then increase to 2-3 leaves.

Ingredients:
- 2 cups zucchini, peeled and cut;
- 1-3 basil leaves;
- 1/2 cup water;

Process:
- Pour water in a small saucepan and add zucchini.
- Bring to a boil, reduce the heat and cook for 10 minutes until water is gone.
- Cool, add basil and blend until smooth.

Pumpkin and apricot puree

This dish looks very tempting especially if you sprinkle it with some pistachios and decorate with chive. It also will be perfect spaghetti sauce.

Ingredients:

- ½ lb peeled pumpkin;
- 6 apricots;
- 1 cup water;

Process:
- Cut the pumpkin into small cubes.
- Wash the apricots, slice them, and remove the stones.
- Put the pumpkin in a pot, pour water, bring to a boil, reduce the heat, and boil for 20 minutes till tender.
- Place the mixture in a blender and blend until smooth. Allow to cool and put into a container. Cover and refrigerate.

Special spinach-potato puree

Ingredients:
- 1/2 lb spinach;
- 1 big or 2 small potatoes;
- 1/2 cup;
- 1 small onion;
- 1 tbsp butter;

Process:
- Peel and chop onion finely.
- Wash spinach thoroughly, dry and chop.
- Peel and cube potato.
- Melt butter in a saucepan with thick bottom, add onion and stew for 4-5 minutes until transparent.
- Add spinach potato and broth and cook for 30-35 minutes over low heat until potato is ready.
- Blend until smooth.

Vegetable broth

You can add any herbs you like. Add dry herbs at the beginning of cooking, and fresh herbs at the end. It's better to remove fresh herbs after 3-5 minutes.

Ingredients:

- 1.1 lb vegetables (carrot, leek, celery stem or roots and sweet pepper);
- 2 l water;
- 1 bay leaf;
- Parsley, thyme or other herbs;
- 4 black peppercorns;
- 1 tbsp oil;

Process:

- Cube all the vegetables.
- Heat oil in a saucepan with thick bottom, add vegetables and stew just for a few minutes (not until golden).
- Add water, freshly ground pepper and bay leaf and cook for about 30 minutes until well cooked.
- Strain the broth.

PORRIDGES

Oatmeal with grapes

For older kids you can add to this recipe an apple and a dried apricot, both cut in small pieces, cinnamon and some honey.

Ingredients:
- 1/3 cup oatmeal;
- 1/5 cup seedless grapes;
- 1 cup water;

Process:
- Grind oatmeal in a coffee grinder
- Pour oatmeal flour in a small saucepan, add hot water slowly, stirring constantly to prevent lumps, then put on the stove and cook over low heat for 5 minutes.
- Wash grapes thoroughly, blend in a blender and pass through a sieve.
- Add grapes to porridge and stir.

Rice porridge with apples and fig

If you keep porridge in the fridge, it becomes too thick, so instead of reheating it, warm it up in a saucepan, adding hot water.

For older kids you can add fresh fruits to porridge.

Ingredients:
- 3/4 cup brown rice flour;
- 2 apples;
- 3-4 dry figs;
- 1 l water;

Process:
- Peel, core and dice the apples and chop the figs finely.
- Pour some water in a saucepan, add fruits and cook over low heat until tender.
- Blend in a blender.
- In another saucepan pour flour and hot water, stirring constantly to prevent lumps, then put on the stove and cook over low heat for 10 minutes.
- Add puree to porridge and stir, until well combined.

HABIT FORMATION

To be honest, I insist on feeding children in a certain hour. If a child has no idea when he will eat, he becomes capricious and nervous.

You also should choose the place to eat. You can't change it every day: kitchen, dining-room, bedroom, bathroom and etc. A child need something stable, he or she needs to know: this is mine, I can be safe here.

And let's not forget about having fun. I chose plates with a bright picture to entertain my children. For example, with Petia we used to play game: he ate something from the plate and I told him: "Look, here we can see a nose. Let's find an ear!" So he never got bored and ate everything well. Or if it doesn't work you can decorate the meal. Use your fantasy!

Mirror, mirror, on the wall….

We want our children to be the best in everything, but the only thing our children want is to be like us. Your child is your reflection. Don't forget about it.

And that is the reason why you should eat with them. You need to show them how to take a spoon, how to hold it and etc. You are a role model and they watch you and repeat after you. That's you should avoid any negative reactions. I mean sometimes we don't like our dinner and we show it. It's unacceptable! You should show only positive emotions towards food.

Also there are a lot of cases when parents enjoy crisps or soda in front of their child and at the same teach him that it's bad and unhealthy to eat something like that. Of course, the child will feel some kind of contradiction. If this food is so unhealthy, why do parents eat it with such a pleasure?

Vegetables

Many parents do the same common mistake – when a baby doesn't drink breast milk anymore, they start giving him different kinds of baby food, which contains much sugar. The baby adjusts to it and later refuses to eat vegetables.

By a year your child's menu should include almost all vegetables, except for legumes, because they are hard to digest, so it's better to give them after two years old and only sometimes, not very often.

Fruits

According to doctors it's better to give fruits in the first half of the day, because they contain much glucose, which makes children more active. To my mind, the best time for fruits is second breakfast. You can make some fruit puree for the whole family, serving it with muesli and yogurt.

Meat products

After a year you can make meatballs, steam patties or a meat soufflé. You can choose any meat you like, for example, my children prefer rabbit meat.

Don't soak meat or fish, otherwise the most part of proteins and minerals will remain in the water. If your child sees little pieces of food and prefers to collect them on the edge of the plate, instead of eating, add smaller pieces into puree every time. It will help your child to adjust to harder foods.

Fish

Give your child fish 1-2 times a week. The best kind for little children is ocean (hake, cod, haddock, salmon, and flounder) and river (trout, silver carp, pike perch) fish. Cook with steam, make sure there is no bones left! If your baby doesn't like fish smell, add some milk to the puree.

One more important thing – fish is a very strong allergen, so you should start with small pieces and watch how the body reacts on it.

Poultry meat

Turkey is the only kind of meat, which doesn't cause any allergies and even boosts immune system. If you want to cook a meat meal for you child, use turkey breast. Forget about meat of goose and duck, till your child is 3 years old. These two types of meat are very hard to digest.

Baking

We all love to treat ourselves with something tasty, and your child is not an exception, so why not to treat him with home baking? It's so easy to make floor at home. You need to buy millet, rinse it with water, dry, grind in a coffee grinder and sift. You can also make floor from white or brown rice, oatmeal or barley.

Approximate daily ration	
Fruit (juice, puree)	200 ml.
Vegetables	0,5 – 0,8 lb.
Porridge	0,3 – 0,5 lb.
Bread	0,1 lb.
Meat	0,1 – 0,2 lb.
Fish	0,05 – 0, 07 lb.
Eggs	1/2
Milk (mixture), kefir	500–600 ml.
Cottage cheese	0,1 lb.
Cheese	0,01 lb.
Sour cream (cream)	0,01 – 0,02 lb.
Butter	0,03 – 0,05 lb.
Vegetable oil	0,01 – 0,02 lb.

1-1.5 YEARS OLD
FRUITS

Fruit yogurt

Fruit yogurt sold in shops contains too much sugar, so it's better to make it by yourself.

Ingredients:
- 1/2 peach, peeled, stone removed;
- 1/2 small banana, peeled;
- 3/5 cup yogurt;
- 2 tsps maple syrup;

Process:
- Cut peach and banana into small pieces.
- Mix all the ingredients and blend in a blender until smooth.

Avocado-banana yogurt

Fruit yogurt sold in shops contains too much sugar, so it's better to make it by yourself.

Ingredients:
- 1/4 avocado, peeled, stone removed;
- 1/2 banana, peeled;
- 2 tbsps yogurt (1 tbsp if it's too thin);

Process:
- Cut avocado and banana into small pieces.
- Add yogurt and blend in a blender until smooth.

Banana- prune puree

Fruit yogurt sold in shops contains too much sugar, so it's better to make it by yourself.

Ingredients:
- 5 prunes;
- 1 small ripe banana, peeled and cut;
- 1 tbsp yogurt

- 1 tbsp cream cheese;

Process:
- Put the prunes in a heatproof bowl and add boiling water to cover. Remove the seed if there are any.
- Mix all the ingredients and blend in a blender until smooth. Add 1-2 tablespoon of fruit juice if necessary.

Tofu with fruit

Ingredients:
- 1 pear;
- 1/2 banana;
- 1/4 cup tufu, cut
- 2/3 cup water;

Process:
- Wash pear and banana thoroughly, peel and cut.
- Pour water in a saucepan, add fruit, bring to a boil and cook over low heat for 5 minutes, until pear is tender.
- Remove from the stove, add tofu, blend in a blender, cool and serve.

Mango and yogurt puree

It's disappointing that mango is not popular today. There are a lot of vitamins, minerals and radical catchers in it, and also there are enzymes which help to improve your digestion and provide relief from heartburn.

Ingredients:
- 1/4 mango;
- 2 tbsps natural yogurt;

Process:
- Wash the mango, slice it, and remove the stones.
- Place the slices and yogurt in a blender and blend until smooth.

Cheese raisin dessert

It's not only healthy, but also delicious!

Ingredients:

- 25g Gruyere cheese (or another hard-pressed cheese);
- ½ apple;
- 15g raisin;
- 1 tbsp natural yogurt;

Process:

- Peel and core the apple, and then grate it.
- Grate the cheese.
- Blend cheese and apple, add raisins and yogurt.

If a child can't chew, it's better to blend all the ingredients in a blender.

Rice with fruit

Ingredients:

- 1 apple;
- 1 peach;
- 1/2 banana
- 1-2 tbsps rice;
- 1 tbsp baby milk or water

Process:

- Grind rice in a coffee grinder
- Cook the apple in a water bath for 5 minutes, then add peach and cook for another 3 minutes.
- Mix apple and peach.
- Mix rice flour with milk or water, add to the puree.

Rice with peaches

Ingredients:

- 1 peach;
- 1 tbsp rice flakes;
- 2/3 cup milk

Process:

- Pour milk in a saucepan, add rice flakes and cook for 5 minutes until thick.
- Peel the peach, cut in half, remove the stone and cut.
- Add peach pieces to porridge.

VEGETABLES

Cabbage surprise

It's a very simple and tasty meal you can serve for lunch. Just multiply all the ingredients and add more grated cheese. Grill or bake in the oven at 355F for 15 minutes.

Ingredients:
- 1,1/2 tbsp brown rice;
- 1 cabbage leaf;
- 1 tomato;
- 1/2 cup parmesan or any hard cheese, grated;
- oil for frying;

Process:
- Cover rice with water and cook for about 25 minutes until done.
- Chop cabbage leaf and cook with steam or in a saucepan, until tender, then drain water.
- Peel tomato, get rid of the seeds and cut.
- Heat some oil in a pan, add tomato, after several minutes add cabbage and simmer for 2 minutes.
- Add grated cheese, stir and cook until cheese melts.
- Mix with rice and cut in pieces.

Tomatoes with carrots and basil

Let your child try new foods to expand your child's palate. Don't be afraid to add herbs, e.g. parsley or basil.

Ingredients:
- 2-3 tomatoes;
- 2-3 cauliflower florets;
- 1 carrot;
- 1/2 cup parmesan or any hard cheese, grated;
- 2-3 fresh basil leaves;
- 1 tbsp butter;

Process:

- Peel the carrot and chop finely, tear up the cauliflower into small florets.
- Pour some water in a small saucepan and cook carrot for 5-10 minutes until done, add florets and cook for another 7-8 minutes. Add water if necessary.
- Peel tomato, get rid of the seeds and chop finely.
- Melt butter in a pan, add tomatoes and simmer until reduced to a thick sauce.
- Add chopped basil and grated cheese.
- Blend carrot and florets in a blender with a small amount of water from the saucepan, than add tomato sauce. Blend sauce if necessary.

Leek, potato and cottage cheese

Ingredients:
- 175g leek;
- 225g potato;
- 2 cup clear vegetable soup;
- 60g cottage cheese;
- 2 tbsps olive oil;

Process:
- Wash the leek, dry and cut thin.
- Peel the potatoes and cut into cubes.
- Preheat a pan, add the olive oil and the leek, and cook for 10 minutes.
- Add potato, pour the soup, cover and simmer for 25030 minutes until done.
- Place the mixture and cottage cheese in a blender and blend until smooth.

Avocado, carrot and cucumber

Adding a little bit of olive oil, lemon juice, pepper and salt will turn this puree into an amazing salad dressing for adults.

Ingredients:
- 1 cup chopped avocado;
- ½ cup peeled and chopped cucumber;
- ¼ cup grated carrot;

- ¼ cup water;
- 3 mint leaves;

Process:

- Place all the ingredients in a blender and blend until smooth.

Zucchini with cheese

Use squash or broccoli instead of zucchini.

Ingredients:

- ½ small zucchini;
- 1 potato;
- 1/2 cup parmesan or any hard cheese, grated;
- 4 tbsps milk;
- 1 tsp butter;

Process:

- Peel the potato and chop finely.
- Pour water in a small saucepan, add potato and cook until done.
- Cut zucchini into slices and cook with steam for 8 minutes.
- Drain water from the saucepan, add butter and grated cheese and stir until well combined.
- Mix all the ingredients and blend until smooth.

Red lentil and apple puree

Ingredients:

- 1 apple;
- 1 ½ cup lentil;
- 2 ½ cup water;

Process:

- Peel the apple and cut.
- Rinse lentil with cold water and pour in a saucepan. Add apple and cover with water.
- Cook for 20-25 minutes.
- Blend until smooth.

Zucchini with tomatoes and pasta stars

Use squash or broccoli instead of zucchini.

Ingredients:

- 3 tomatoes;
- 1/2 small zucchini;
- 2 tbsps cheddar, grated;
- 2 tbsps pasta stars;
- 1 1/2 tbsp butter;

Process:

- Cook the pasta according to package direction.
- Peel tomato, get rid of the seeds and cut.
- Peel and dice zucchini.
- Melt butter in a pan, add zucchini and simmer for 5 minutes.
- Add tomatoes and cook over medium heat for another 5 minutes.
- Remove from the stove, add grated cheese and stir until cheese melts.
- Blend in a blender until smooth, and then stir with pasta.

Cauliflower with cheese

Drop the last point for older children.

Ingredients:

- 0,4 lb cauliflower;
- 2/3 milk;
- 2 tbsps parmesan or any hard cheese, grated;
- 1 tbsp butter;
- 1 tbsp flour;

Process:

- Rinse cauliflower thoroughly, tear up into small florets and cook with steam for 10 minutes, until done.
- Melt butter in a saucepan with thick bottom; add flour, stirring gently to prevent lumps.
- Add milk, whisking constantly. Cook over low heat, whisking, until smooth.

- Cook the pasta according to package direction.
- Remove from the stove and add cheese. Keep stirring, until cheese melts.
- Add the sauce to cauliflower and blend until smooth.

Risotto with pumpkin

Ingredients:
- 0,7 lb cauliflower;
- 0,4 lb rice for risotto;
- 1/2 l vegetable broth;
- 1 small onion;
- 1 garlic clove;
- 4 tbsps parmesan or any hard cheese, grated;
- 2 tbsps butter;
- 2 tbsps cream;
- handful parsley, finely chopped;
- olive oil;
- sea salt;

Process:
- Preheat oven to 390F.
- Peel, remove the core and cut pumpkin into small cubes. Drizzle with olive oil and sprinkle with sea salt. Bake for 20 minutes until golden.
- Peel onion and garlic and chop finely.
- Melt butter in a pan, add onion and garlic, cook until transparent.
- Add rice and cook for 2-3 minutes.
- Add a half cup of hot broth, as the rice slowly absorbs the liquid it's in. Keep adding the same amount of the broth, until you run out of it. Cook for 15-18 minutes.
- Add pumpkin, parsley, grated cheese and cream and stir.

Vichyssoise

Ingredients:

- 1 small shallot;
- 2 leeks (only green part);
- 3 medium potatoes;
- 600 ml vegetable broth
- 2 tbsps low fat sour cream or yogurt;
- oil for frying;
- some parsley and chive for garnish;

Process:

- Chop shallot and leeks finely.
- Pour some oil in saucepan and add shallot and leeks. Stew for 5 minutes.
- Peel and cut potatoes.
- Add potatoes and broth to the saucepan and cook until done.
- Set soup aside for some time to cool, then beat until smooth and add sour cream or yogurt.
- Garnish with cut parsley and chive

Celery root and carrot soup

Ingredients:

- 0,7 lb celery root;
- 1 small onion;
- 0,7 lb carrot;
- 800 ml vegetable broth
- 1 garlic clove;
- 1 bay leaf;
- parsley, chopped, to your taste;
- 1 tbsp olive oil;

Process:

- Chop onion and garlic finely.

- Pour oil in saucepan with thick bottom, and add onion and garlic. Stew for several minutes.
- Dice celery root and carrot, add to the saucepan and cook for 3-4 minutes.
- Pour the hot broth in, add bay leaf and cook until celery root is tender.
- Remove the bay leaf, add parsley and beat until well combined.

Potatoes with parsnip and rabbit meat

If you want to froze it, make puree when all the vegetables are cold.

Ingredients:
- 0,2 lb boiled rabbit meat;
- 0,2 lb potato;
- 3 tbsps parship, chopped;
- 1 ½ tbsp green beans, chopped;
- 4 tbsps milk;

Process:
- Wash potato and parsnip thoroughly, peel and chop.
- Cut off the ends of green beans.
- Put all the vegetables in a saucepan, cover with water, bring to a boil, cover and cook over low heat until tender.
- Drain water, blend the vegetables, rabbit meat and milk in a blender until smooth.

1.5-3 years old

Fruits

Green fruit salad

Ingredients:
- 0,3 lb green grapes;
- 2 kiwis;
- 1 green apple;
- 1 small green watermelon;
- 100 ml tepid water;
- 2 tsps powdered sugar or maple syrup;

Process:
- Wash, peel and cut all fruit.
- Pour powdered sugar in a cup and add water, stirring constantly.
- Season fruit salad with sweet water. You can use lemon or any other fruit juice instead, if it tastes too sweet.

Dried apricot with papaya and pear

Ingredients:
- 8-10 dried apricots;
- ½ ripe papaya;
- 1 ripe juicy pear;

Process:
- Peel papaya and pear, remove the core and cut in small pieces.
- Rinse dried apricots with water, put in a small saucepan and cover with water. Bring to a boil and cook over low heat for 8 minutes until tender.
- Cut dried apricots and mix with papaya and pear. Blend in a blender if your child prefers soft foods.

Ginger syrup

Ingredients:
- 1 ginger;
- 3 tbsps sugar;

Process:
- Peel and grate the ginger.
- Add sugar and water, bring to a boil.
- Pour syrup through a sieve, discard ginger.

Quince marmalade

This dessert is somewhere between jam and puree. If there are some lumps, you may blend the mixture in a blender. It's also possible to use it instead of sugar in puree.

Ingredients:

- 200g quince;
- 100g sugar;

Process:
- Wash the quince, cut it in halves and core it.
- Cut into cubes, add sugar and water, and bring to a boil.
- Reduce the heat, and stir for 10 minutes. Then bring to a boil again. Repeat for 3 times.

Swiss fruit muesli

Ingredients:
- 3 tbsp oat flakes;
- 2 tsps wheat germ;
- 1 apple;
- 1 pear;
- 1 tsp maple syrup;
- 120-150 ml yogurt;
- 175 ml apple juice;
- 1 tsp lemon juice;

Process:
- Mix oat flakes and wheat germ with apple juice and put in the fridge for several hours or for a night.
- Peel and grate the apple.
- Peel the pear, remove the core and chop finely.
- Mix apple and lemon juice.
- Add oat flakes and wheat germ, pear, maple syrup and yogurt and stir until well combined.

Flakes breakfast

Ingredients:
- ½ cup of any flakes (oat, rye, buckwheat);
- 1 small banana;
- 3 tbsps yogurt or milk;

Process:
- Peel banana and chop finely.
- Crush flakes in a mortar, add banana and stir well.
- Add yogurt or milk, stir again and serve.

Home muesli

Ingredients:
- 2 tbsps oat flakes for fast cooking;
- 1 tbsp raisin;
- 1 apple;
- 2 tbsps cottage cheese;
- ½ tsp sesame seeds;
- 1 tsp liquid honey;
- juice of half a lemon;

Process:
- Cover oat flakes with a small amount of hot water.
- Put raisins in a bowl and pour in warm water.
- Grate apple on a coarse grater and drizzle with lemon juice.
- Mix all the ingredients, stir well and serve.

VEGETABLES

Apple and vegetables and lentil puree

Ingredients:

- 1 ½ medium carrot;
- 3-4 tbsps red lentil, ground;
- 350 ml vegetable broth or water;
- 2-3 cauliflower florets;
- ½ apple;
- 0,2 lb leek;
- 2 tbsps butter;

Process:

- Wash onion thoroughly and chop.
- Melt butter in a saucepan and stew onion for 5 minutes.
- Peel and cut carrots, then add to onion and cook for 2-3 minutes.
- Add lentil and broth, bring to a boil, cover and cook over low heat for 10 minutes.
- Tear up the cauliflower into small florets.
- Peel the apple, remove the core and chop.
- Add cauliflower and apple to the saucepan and cook for 15 minutes until done.
- Blend in a blender until smooth.

Lentil with vegetables

Add more vegetable broth to get a soup for the whole family.

Ingredients:

- ½ shallot;
- 1 carrot;
- ½ celery;
- ½ yam;
- 400 ml vegetable broth or water;
- 2 tbsps red lentil;

- 1 tbsps olive oil;

Process:
- Peel and chop onion, carrot, celery and yam finely. Don't mix.
- Heat oil in a saucepan with thick bottom, add onion and stew for several minutes until transparent.
- Add carrot and celery and stew for 5 minutes until tender.
- Add lentil and yam. Pour in broth or water, bring to a boil, reduce the heat, cover and cook for 20 minutes until done.
- Blend in a blender.

Green pea puree

The best thing about green pea is that it doesn't need salt, sugar or any other seasonings.

Ingredients:
- 1 cup frozen peas;
- 1 cup water;

Process:
- Pour water in a pot, add peas, and bring to a boil.
- Reduce the heat, and boil for 15 minutes until done.
- Place in a blender and blend until smooth.

Carrot and chickpea puree

If you fail to find chickpea in groceries, you can use dry pea.

Ingredients:
- ½ cup washed and peeled carrot;
- 1 cup dry pea;
- 1 cup water;

Process:
- Soak the peas for the night. In the morning drain the water and rinse the peas.
- Put the peas in a pot, cover with water and boil for 45 minutes.
- Add the carrot and boil for another 15 minutes.

- Place in a blender and blend until smooth.

Lentil and chicken puree

Ingredients:
- ¾ cup red lentil;
- 1 medium piece of skinless chicken breast;
- 1 cup water;

Process:
- Rinse lentil with cold water.
- Wash chicken breast thoroughly; dry with a paper towel and dice.
- Put lentil and chicken in the saucepan, cover with water, bring to a boil, reduce the heat, and cook for 25 minutes until done.
- Blend in a blender.

Sweet vegetable puree

Ingredients:
- ½ medium onion;
- 1 medium carrot;
- 2 small potatoes;
- 2 tbsps fresh or frozen corn;
- 1 tbsp fresh or frozen green peas;
- 200 ml water;
- 1 tbsp olive oil;

Process:
- Chop all the vegetables finely, except corn and pea.
- Heat olive oil in a pan and fry onion over low heat until tender.
- Add carrot and cook for 5 minutes.
- Put fried onion and carrot in a saucepan, add potato and water, bring to a boil, cover and cook over low heat for 10-15 minutes, until potato is tender.
- Add corn and pea, cook for another 2 minutes.
- Blend in a blender and pass through a sieve.

Green fingers

Ingredients:

- 0,4 lb green beans;
- 1 small onion;
- 2 medium tomatoes;
- ½ tbsp tomato paste;
- 1 ½ hard cheese, grated;
- 1 tbsp butter;

Process:

- Peel onion and chop finely.
- Melt butter in a pan and cook onion for 4 minutes, until tender, but not golden.
- Cut off the ends of green beans, put in a saucepan, cover with water and cook for 6-8 minutes.
- Peel tomatoes, remove the seeds, chop finely and mix with onion, tomato pasta and cheese.
- Cover green beans with the sauce.

White bean and veal puree

White bean puree can be a great sauce if you add some horseradish, garlic and salad oil in it. You can serve it with vegetables or meat.

Ingredients:

- ½ cup dry white bean;
- ¾ cup chopped carrot;
- 125g veal tenderloin;
- 3 cup water;

Process:

- Soak the beans for the night.
- In the morning drain the water and rinse the peas.
- Put the peas in a pot, cover with 3 cup water and boil until tender.
- Add the chopped veal, and boil for another 20 minutes until done.
- Add the carrot and boil for 10 minutes.
- Place in a blender and blend until smooth.

Vegetables with cheese sauce

Ingredients:
- 2-3 cauliflower florets;
- 1 carrot;
- 2 tbps frozen green peas;
- ½ small zucchini;

Cheese sauce:
- 2 tbsp butter;
- 2 tbsps flour;
- 1 cup milk;
- 3 tbsps hard cheese, grated;

Process:
- Tear up the cauliflower into small florets.
- Peel carrot and slice thinly.
- Slice zucchini.
- Cook carrot and cauliflower with steam for 6 minutes, add peas and zucchini and cook for another 4 minutes, until tender.
- Cut all the vegetables or make a puree. Serve with cheese sauce.

Cheese sauce:
- Melt butter, mix with flour and fry it for 2-3 minutes.
- Add milk, stirring constantly and cook over medium heat, until smooth. Bring to a boil and cook for 1 minute, stirring.
- Remove from the stove; add cheese, stirring, until cheese melts.

Roasted garlic

This recipe originally belongs to Thailand. Roasted garlic is sliced in halves and served as butter. You can eat it with bread or cereals. It has unique and really unusual taste.

Ingredients:
- 1 garlic bulb;

Process:
- Preheat your oven to 350F.
- Peel the garlic, and trim the top of it.
- Wrap in foil and place to the oven. Roast for 40 minutes.
- Let the garlic cool and add it to different sauces and dishes.

Cauliflower, paprika and corn puree

Children enjoy the bright colours and amazing taste of these vegetables! So don't hesitate to try.

Ingredients:
- 100g cauliflower;
- 25g bell pepper;
- 75g fresh or frozen corn;
- ½ cup milk;
- 50g grated parmesan cheese;

Process:
- Cut the cauliflower into florets and boil in a pot with milk for 8 minutes until tender.
- Add grated cheese and stir until melted.
- Corn and chopped bell pepper boil in a pot for 6-8 minutes. Then drain water, dry the vegetables with a paper towel, place them in a blender and blend until smooth.
- Add boiled cauliflower, milk and blend again.

Green bean and basil puree

You can blend bean and potato puree to please elder children. If a child doesn't like basil you can replace it with parsley. Don't be afraid of experiments – there are a lot of radical catchers in herbs. They boost your immune system.

Ingredients:
- 1 ½ cup green bean;
- 1 tbsp chopped basil;
- 1 cup water;

Process:

- Boil the beans until tender. Drain the water in another pot, and place the beans in a container with ice.
- Place beans and basil into a blender and blend until smooth. Add water if needed.

Pistou sauce (fennel and apple sauce)

Pistou sauce is very famous kind of sauce in Nice. Usually there are no any herbs in it, but it's better to change it a little bit for children. You can serve it with spaghetti or cream soup.

Ingredients:
- 1 fennel, sliced;
- 1 apple, sliced;
- 1 clove garlic, roasted (p. 119)
- bunch of parsley, chopped;
- 1 scallion leaf, chopped;
- 1 cup water;
- 2 tbsps olive oil;

Process:
- Put sliced apple and fennel in a pit, and boil until tender.
- Place chopped parsley, scallion, roasted garlic, olive oil, boiled apple and fennel in a blender, and blend until smooth.

SOUP

Broccoli soup

Ingredients:

- 1 carrot;
- 1 potato;
- 150g peeled pumpkin;
- 150-200g florets broccoli;
- 2 cups broth;
- 1 cup milk;
- 1 tbsp olive oil;
- 1 tbsp butter;
- 1 onion;
- 1 clove garlic;

Process:

- Put the butter and olive oil in a preheated pan, add garlic and onion and cook for 5 minutes until tender.
- Add chopped vegetables and cook for 3 minutes.
- Pour hot broth and bring to a boil. Reduce the heat, cover and cook for another 20 minutes until tender.
- Place in a blender, add milk and blend until smooth.

Minestrone

You can add alphabet spaghetti to please you child. Adults will enjoy this soup even more if you serve it with roasted garlic bread.

Ingredients:

- 50g carrot;
- 50g potato;
- 1 onion, chopped;
- 50 leek (white part), chopped;

- 50g tomatoes;
- 50g green beans;
- 50g frozen peas;
- 1 clove garlic, chopped;
- basil or parsley;
- 3-4 cup broth (p. 54);
- 1 tbsp olive oil;

Process:
- Cook onion, leek and garlic in a preheated pan.
- To peel tomatoes gently place them into boiling water and boil for 25-30 seconds (not more). Then place them into a boil with iced water and let them cool off. After peeling cut tomatoes in small cubes.
- Peel carrot and potato and cut into cubes too.
- Place the vegetables in a pot, pour the broth, bring to a boil, then reduce the heat and boil for 5 minutes.
- Add green beans and frozen peas and boil for another 5 minutes. You can sprinkle it with basil or parsley or add grated cheese.

Green peas soup

It's better to use shallot not to spoil delicate flower of green peas.

Ingredients:
- 300g frozen peas;
- 1 shallot, chopped;
- 2 cups broth (p. 54);
- ½ cup natural yogurt or sour cream;
- mint;
- olive oil;

Process:
- Cook the onion for 3 minutes in a skillet.

- Add peas, mint and pour hot broth. Bring to a boil, reduce the heat and cook until the peas are tender.
- Puree in a blender.
- Add yogurt or sour cream and mint.

Pea and zucchini soup

You can turn it into soup for the whole family by adding seasonings and increasing the amount of ingredients.

Ingredients:
- 50g zucchini, peeled and sliced;
- 150g potato, peeled and cut into cubes;
- 25g frozen peas;
- 1 small onion, chopped;
- ½ cup vegetable broth (p. 54);
- 1 tbsp butter;

Process:
- Cook the onion in a skillet until tender in some butter.
- Add sliced zucchini, potato and broth. Bring to a boil, then cover and cook over low heat for 12 minutes.
- Pour frozen peas, bring to a boil again, then reduce the heat and cook for another 5 minutes.
- Place everything in a blender and blend until smooth.

Creamy chicken soup with celeriac and potato

Ingredients:
- 2 boneless chicken breasts;
- ½ celeriac (chopped);
- 2 potatoes (peeled and chopped);
- 1 clove garlic, roasted (p. 119);
- 2 cup water;
- 1 tsp butter;

- sea salt;

Process:

- Wash chicken breasts, dry them with a towel, and cut into cubes.
- Melt the butter in a pan, and add roasted garlic, chicken, potatoes and celeriac. Cook for 5 minutes, stirring occasionally.
- Pour the water, sprinkle with salt and bring to a boil. Reduce the heat, cover and cook for 10-15 minutes.
- Put everything in a blender and blend until smooth.

GROATS

Fresh pear and semolina

Instead pear you can use apricots or apple puree with cinnamon.

Ingredients:
- 1 tbsp semolina;
- ½ cup milk;
- 1 fresh pear, peeled and cored;
- 2 tsps maple syrup;
- 1 pinch cinnamon;

Process:
- Cut the pear into cubes.
- Boil milk in a pot over low heat, pour semolina and boil constantly stirring. Bring to a boil and boil for another 2 minutes.
- Add the pear, maple syrup, cinnamon and puree in a blender.
- It's possible not to blend the pear – just cut it into cubes and add to the porridge.

Buckwheat and tofu

Ingredients:
- 100g buckwheat;
- 1 pack tofu;
- 1 root ginger;
- 1 clove garlic, minced;
- ¼ tsp nutmeg;
- 1 tsp dried basil;
- 1 bunch of fresh basil;
- 1 cup hot water;
- 1 tsp olive oil;
- 2 tbsps soy sauce;

Process:

- Grate the ginger.
- Cook the ginger, garlic, nutmeg and soy sauce in the olive oil aboth 2 minutes.
- Add buckwheat and continue cooking over a medium-low heat for 7 minutes.
- Pour water, cover and cook over a low heat for 12-15 minutes.
- Add dried basil, making sure to stir well.
- Serve the dish with tofu and leaves of fresh basil.

Buckwheat and vegetables

If your children get bored with buckwheat, surprise them with this recipe.

Ingredients:
- 1 cup buckwheat;
- 1 zucchini, peeled and sliced;
- 1 red onion, peeled and sliced;
- 2 cup water;
- 1 tsp balsamic vinegar;
- 1 tbsp Narsharab sauce;
- 1 tbsp olive oil;
- fresh cilantro or parsley;
- sea salt;

Process:
- Grill zucchini and onion.
- Boil buckwheat in a pot with water, bring to a boil, add salt, reduce the heat, cover and cook until done.
- Chop the grilled vegetables and mix with buckwheat.
- Combine olive oil, Narsharab sauce and balsamic vinegar in a bowl.
- Add the mixture to the buckwheat and serve warm.

Couscous

Couscous is extremely underrated! We feed our children with semolina though couscous is also healthy and delicious wheat.

Ingredients:
- 45g couscous;
- 1 bell pepper, chopped;
- 1 tomato, peeled and chopped;
- scallion;
- 1 tbsp raisin;
- 1 tbsp cedar nuts;
- ½ cup vegetable broth (p. 54);

For salad dressing:
- 1 tbsp olive oil;
- 1 tsp balsamic vinegar;
- ½ tsp clear honey;

Process:
- Cook couscous following the directions on a package using the broth instead of water.
- Combine chopped tomato, belly pepper and cooked couscous together.
- Mix olive oil, balsamic vinegar and honey and combine with the couscous. Sprinkle with cedar nuts, raisins and chopped scallion and serve warm.

EGGS AND COTTAGE CHEESE

Scrambled eggs

It's better to avoid excessive eggs consumption, but my children really enjoy this recipe so sometimes I indulge them.

Ingredients:
- 4 eggs;
- 50g cheese;
- parsley or basil;

Process:
- Preheat your oven to 340F.
- Separate the white from the yolk.
- Beat the white eggs until stiff and place on the roasting dish.
- Make hollows and place the yolks in them.
- Cook in the oven until done.
- Sprinkle with cheese and basil or parsley.

Eggs cooked in Bain Marie

Eggs should be fresh. If your child prefers medium-timed eggs, it's better to cook them less than 5 minutes. You can use cream, but sour cream is preferable.

Ingredients:
- 5 eggs;
- 5 tsps sour cream;
- sea salt;
- freshly ground black pepper;

Process:
- Preheat your oven to 340F.
- Oil ceramic baking molds.
- Crack an egg into every mold, add 1 tsp sour cream and sprinkle with salt and peer to taste.
- Pour hot water in a baking dish and place molds with eggs in it. Cook for 7-8 minutes.
- Serve with roasted garlic rye-bread.

Parmentier eggs

It's very easy and interesting to cook, and usually both children and adults enjoy it.

Ingredients:
- 2 potatoes, peeled and sliced into halves;
- 4 eggs;
- 100g Gruyere cheese;
- 2 tsps butter;
- olive oil;
- freshly ground black pepper;
- sea salt;

Process:
- Remove the core of each potato with a spoon, and trim the lowest part of the half to make potato stable.
- Place the potatoes into a pot with boiling salted water for 2-3 minutes. Then dry them with a paper towel and drizzle with olive oil. Don't forget to sprinkle with salt.
- Place the halves on the roasting dish and roast in the oven until golden brown.
- Wrap the halves in a foil (leave the top unwrapped), put them on the roasting dish again and crack the eggs into the hollows.
- Sprinkle with salt and pepper. Also you can sprinkle it with grated cheese and add 1 tsp of butter.
- Place in the oven and cook for 2-3 minutes until eggs are done.

Carrot curd croquets

Ingredients:
- 400g curd;
- 1 apple;
- 1 carrot;
- 1 egg;
- 1 tbsp sugar;
- 3 tbsps flour;

- olive oil;
- sea salt;

Process:
- Preheat your oven to 340F.
- Peel and grate the carrot and the apple, and combine with curd.
- Add sugar, a little bit of salt, 2 tbsps flour, and egg and mix well.
- Form the croquets, sprinkle with flour, and fry on both sides.
- Place on a baking sheet and cook in the oven until done.

Curd croquets with cherry sauce

Add a tablespoon of cherry liqueur to make the taste of the sauce better.

Ingredients:
- 300g curd;
- 1 egg;
- ½ cup frozen cherries;
- 1 tsp starch;
- 2 tbsp sugar;
- 1 tbsp cold water;
- a pinch of cinnamon;
- 1 tbsp sour cream;
- olive oil;
- sea salt;

Process:
- Combine the curd, egg, 1 tbsp sugar and salt in a bowl and mix well.
- Form the croquets, sprinkle with flour, and fry on both sides in a pan.
- Place the pan with the croquets in an oven until done.
- To make the sauce place the frozen cherries in a pan, add sugar and starch diluted with water. Sprinkle the mixture with cinnamon and then bring to a boil stirring occasionally. Continue the cooking until the sauce is quite thick.
- Serve the croquets with cherry sauce and sour cream.

Fruit curd dessert with bread

Ingredients:

- 500g curd;
- 1 ½ cup sour cream;
- 300g rye bread;
- a handful of prune;
- 2/3 cup sugar;
- 5-6 apples;
- cinnamon to taste;

Process:

- Rub the curd through a tammy, add the sour cream and 1/3 cup sugar and mix well.
- Grate the rye bread.
- Peel and core the apples, cut them into cubes.
- To cook sugar liqueur pour sugar diluted with water in a pot. Cook it over medium heat stirring occasionally until melt. Add chopped prunes and bring to a boil.
- Add apples and cinnamon and cook until tender.
- Place the curd in a coupe with layers of bread, apples and prunes.

BAKING

Pearl bread

You can use graham flour mixed with rye flour instead of the pearl one.

Ingredients:
- 120g pearl barley;
- 250g pearl flour (p. 42);
- 20g fresh yeast;
- 1 cup warm water;
- ¼ tsp grated nutmeg;
- 1 tsp sea salt;

Process:
- Preheat your oven to 480F.
- Give the barley a quick rinse before the cooking.
- Boil the pearl barley over low heat until tender.
- Pour warm water in a bowl, add yeast and stir until melted. Then add the flour, mix well.
- Add the pearl barley to the pastry, sprinkle with the grated nutmeg and mix well. Leave for 40 minutes in a warm place.
- Oil a roasting dish, place the mixture in it and leave for another 15 minutes.
- Cook in the preheated oven for 40 minutes. Then open the oven door and cook for another 10 minutes.

French toasts

Ingredients:
- 1 egg;
- 2 tbsps milk;
- 2 loaves of bread;
- 25g butter;
- a pinch of cinnamon;

Process:

- Beat up the egg and milk in a bowl, sprinkle with cinnamon.
- Dip the loaves in the mixture.
- Fry the loaves in butter until golden brown.
- Serve with maple syrup or jam.

Raisin nut cookies

Ingredients:
- 2 cups chestnut or buckwheat flour;
- 1 cup raisin;
- ½ cup cedar nuts;
- ½ chopped walnuts;
- 2 tbsps olive oil;
- 2 ½ cup warm water;
- 1 rosemary sprig;
- 2 tbsps sugar;
- a pinch of sea salt;

Process:
- Preheat your oven to 320F.
- Put flour through a sieve, add 1 ½ cup water, 1 tbsp olive oil, sugar and salt and mix well. Leave for an hour.
- Place the raisins in a bowl, cover them with warm water and leave for 20 minutes. Then dry with a paper towel.
- Oil a baking dish.
- Roll out the dough and place it in the baking dish.
- Sprinkle it with raisins, nuts and chopped rosemary.
- Bake in the oven for 40 minutes and then cut into cubes.

Strawberry rice pudding

The main tip for cooking pudding is to do it slowly and very carefully. Start cooking right after breakfast and it will be done for lunch.

Ingredients:
- 50g rice;
- ½ tsp vanilla essence;
- 1 ½ tsp powdered sugar;
- 2 ½ cup milk;
- butter;
- strawberry jam;

Process:
- Preheat your oven to 300F.
- Combine rice, milk, vanilla essence and powdered sugar and mix well.
- Place the mixture in an oiled baking dish and put the butter in the middle. Bake in the preheated oven for 1 ½ - 2 hours stirring occasionally.
- Serve with strawberry jam.

FROM 3 TO 7

Since 3 years old a child starts studying the world around him. His mind is widely open and he is ready to learn new things.

Once my son and I had a walk and found a leaf of myrtle – an amazing plant with beautiful leaves. I rubbed the leaf and said: "Here! Smell it!" Some days later I saw my son rubbing something with his friend – she is a little bit younger than he – and I heard how he told her: "Here! Smell it!"

Children are very sensitive to the information you give them. It's very important for them and we can use it to open their heads about the world and… food!

Taste of joy

In the period of 3 to 6 years taste buds develop and it's very important not to miss it and show different kinds of seasonings to your child. I have a friend who was sure that a child didn't need to know any seasonings at all. So she didn't add them until he went to school. And when she decided to show him parsley and fennel he didn't even want to try them. In fact, now her son avoids any kind of herbs.

Don't make such a mistake. Add different types of herbs to everything: meat, soup, fish and etc. The best herbs for children are parsley, basil, cilantro, fennel, thyme, oregano, and scallion. All of them contain important vitamins and minerals.

Garden on your window sill

To make a child get used to herbs you can grow them on your window sill. Buy a pot, place it on the window sill and cast any seeds you like. You can buy everything needed in every supermarket. Also it can show to your child how it is important and responsible to take care of something. And definitely he will want to try the fruits of his labour.

Home diplomacy

My husband used to tell me that if he had refused to eat everything up, he would have been kept hungry until evening. His siblings got the dessert or some fruits, but he was told: "You didn't finish your meal so you are not hungry."

Sounds tough but I think it has a point. No one wants to offend or insult a child! He was directly told: "If you don't want, fine!" But you will receive next meal only in prescribed time. Because if a kind granny gives the child something tasty after that, he will miss the next dinner too! He will be sure that his granny will feed him so what is the point to eat soup when you can have a cake later?

It is necessarily to learn how to come to an agreement with your child. There is no need to alter the character of the child, just show him that there are frames and rules he must follow. It will make him stronger and more flexible in future.

No TV!

Some may not agree but I am sure that until 4 a child shouldn't even know about TV. This flood of information prevents the development of a child and his self-expression.

Strict regime

My children have rather strict regime. At 8am they have breakfast, at noon – lunch, at 5pm – dinner, at 7pm – supper. This schedule never changes. Of course, when we are on the trip or someone is ill, the schedule changes a bit, but then it comes back. My husband and I have a crazy regime so sometimes I can have breakfast only at 11am or eat just once a day. But it doesn't reflect on children. 8am, noon, 5pm, 7pm – always!

Daycare

When a child turns three parents don't know whether their child should stay at home or go into daycare. A lot of mother cares about menu, about the healthiness of the food. No need to worry. Children's diet is well planned and calculated. A child must get meat or fish, vegetables, fruits and milk products. And there is a strict control over this diet.

Approximate daily ration for 3-6 years old child

Fruits	230-250g
Vegetables	230-250g
Potato	100-150g
Grits and macaroni products	40g
Bread	100g
Meat	110-120g
Fish	<40g
Eggs	½ in a day or 1 in two days
Milk and cultured milk foods	500-600ml
Curd	50g
Cheese	10g
Butter	30g
Salad oil	10-15

3-6 YEARS OLD SALADS

Steamed vegetable salad

You can use both fresh and steamed vegetables for your salad.

Ingredients:

- Broccoli;
- Cauliflower;
- Brussels sprouts;
- Carrot;

Process:

- Cut the broccoli and cauliflower into florets.
- Peel the carrot and cut it into slices.
- Steam the vegetables, place them into a bowl and dress the salad.

Fresh vegetable salad

Ingredients:

- Celeriac;
- Carrot;
- Garden radish;
- Cucumber;
- Leaves of lettuce;

Process:

- Tear the leaves of lettuce into pieces.
- Cut the cucumber and garden radish.
- Peel and grate the celeriac and carrot.
- Combine all the ingredients and dress the salad.

Salad dressing

Ingredients:
- 1 tbsp baby yogurt;
- 1 tbsp sour cream;
- 1 tbsp lemon juice;
- 2 tbsp cold milk;
- 1 garlic clove (finely chopped);
- 1 tsp tomato paste;
- 1 tbsp cheese (finely grated);

Process:
- Combine the yogurt and sour cream.
- Add lemon juice, milk, garlic; tomato paste and cheese.
- Mix well.

Chinese cucumber salad

If your children don't like sesame, you can replace it with almond or some nut oil. If don't have any, you can melt some butter and use it as dressing. But eat warm.

Ingredients:
- 1 carrot;
- 1 cucumber;
- ½ apple;
- Sesame seeds;
- 1 tsp soy sauce;
- 1 tbsp salad oil;
- 1 tbsp honey or maple syrup;
- 1 tsp gingili oil;

Process:
- Grate the carrot, cucumber and apple, mix well and place into a bowl.
- Combine the soy sauce, salad and gingili oil, honey or maple syrup.
- Dress the salad and sprinkle it with sesame.

Hawaiian salad with chicken

Children enjoy this salad, because it's sweet and tasty. But don't forget that canned pineapple and corn should be preservative-free and have minimum percentage of sugar.

Ingredients:

- 100g Basmati rice;
- 1 boneless and skinless chicken breast;
- 2 tbsps frozen green peas;
- 2 tbsps canned corn;
- ¼ fresh pineapple or ½ canned pineapple;
- 1 tomato;
- Salad oil;
- 1 tsp lemon juice;
- Potherb;

Process:

- Boil rice according to the instruction on the pack.
- Boil the chicken breast and then cut it into cubes.
- Put the frozen green peas into boiled water for 3 minutes and then put into ice. It will help to keep the form and color of peas.
- Cut the pineapple into cubes.
- Combine all the ingredients.
- Combine pineapple and lemon juice and salad oil. Dress the salad and sprinkle it with potherbs.

SOUPS

Pumpkin soup with orange

Ingredients:
- 300-400g pumpkin;
- 600-800mL clear vegetable soup;
- 1 onion;
- ½ cup orange juice;
- ½ tsp orange zest;
- Cilantro;
- 1 tbsp salad oil;
- Sour cream;

Process:
- Peel and cut the pumpkin.
- Chop the onion.
- Cook the onion on preheated frying pan for 3 minutes. Add the pumpkin, cook for 1 more minute, and pour the vegetable soup. Bring to a boil and cook over low heat for 15-20 minutes.
- Cool the soup, add orange juice and zest, cilantro and blend until smooth.

Before serving add 1 tsp sour cream.

Carrot and lentils soup

There are a lot healthy elements in lentils: iron, zinc, and etc.

Ingredients:
- 4 tbsps lentils;
- 400g carrot;
- 1 leek;
- 300ml milk;
- 1 tbsp olive oil;
- 600 hot water or clear vegetable soup;
- ½ tsp grated coriander seeds;

- Sea salt;
- Freshly ground pepper;

Process:
- Heat the oil in a frying pan. Add chopped white part of the leek and cook for 3 minutes.
- Add dry lentils, carrot cut into cubes, coriander seeds, and let it soak in oil.
- Pour hot water or vegetable soup, lower the heat, cover and cook for 20 minutes.
- The ¼ of the porridge blend until smooth.
- Place back into the pan, add milk, add sea salt and pepper to taste.

Hot meal

Zucchini boats

Every child has that very period when he hates vegetables. And there is a great way to hide them!

Ingredients:
- 1 zucchini;
- 1 sweet pepper;
- 1 egg;
- 1 tbsp milk;
- 60g ground rusks;
- 4 tbsps finely grated cheese;
- 1 tbsp flour;
- Olive oil;
- Sea salt;
- Freshly ground pepper;

Process:
- Preheat the oven to 340F.
- Cut the zucchini into half, remove the core and cut it.
- Whip eggs with milk.
- Add ground rusks, chopped zucchini and grated cheese to the eggs. Add salt and pepper.
- Roll the halves of the zucchini in flour and fry until golden crust.
- Put the feeling in a hollow of the fried zucchini.

- Remove the peduncle of the sweet pepper, seeds and slice into 4 pieces.
- Make the sails using pepper and toothpicks.
- Sprinkle the boats with olive oil, put them into oven and cook for 10-15 minutes until tender.

Vegetable cutlets

Ingredients:
- 1 medium potato;
- 1 medium carrot;
- 1 red onion;
- ¼ leek (white part);
- 1 glove garlic;
- 50g mushrooms;
- 70g cheese;
- 1 egg;
- 1 yolk;
- 1 tbsp soy sauce;
- 2 tbsps olive oil;
- Salad oil;
- 3 tbsps flour;
- 100g ground rusks;
- ½ tsp thyme;
- Sea salt;
- Freshly ground pepper;

Process:
- Preheat the oven to 340F.
- Wash the mushrooms and slice them. Onion, leek and garlic chop finely, but don't combine.
- Grate the carrot.
- Boil unpeeled potato until cooked (for 25 minutes), peel it, grate and add some olive oil.
- Heat 1 tbsp salad oil, fry the onion and garlic, add grated carrot, leek, mushrooms, thyme and stew for 10 minutes over medium heat

- Combine stewed vegetables with grated potato, cheese, 25g rusks, soy sauce, and yolk. Add salt and pepper to taste and mix well.
- Make 12-15 small patties, roll them in flour, then in beaten egg, and in ground rusks.
- Fry patties in a pan a little bit and then place them into preheated oven for 10 minutes.

Vegetable kebab

Ingredients:
- Sweet peppers of different colors;
- Zucchini;
- Carrot;
- Other vegetables on your taste;
- Olive oil;
- Balsamic vinegar;
- Honey;

Process:
- Cut the vegetables into cubes. Combine olive oil, balsamic vinegar and honey.
- Add the sauce to the vegetables. Put them on a stick and place into the preheated oven. Bake until done.

Ratatouille

Ingredients:
- 2 eggplants;
- 2 zucchinis;
- 2 carrots;
- 1 sweet pepper;
- 1 apple;
- 1 onion;
- 1 glove garlic;
- Olive oil;
- Cider vinegar;

Process:
- Peel the carrot, remove the peduncle and seeds of the sweet pepper. Also remove eggplant's peduncle.
- Cut all the ingredients into cubes and place them into earthenware.
- Add 1 tbsp olive oil, cover and stew in the oven for 30 minutes. You can add cider vinegar if you want.

Spanish omelet

Ingredients:
- 4 eggs;
- 2 potatoes;
- 1 tomato;
- 2 onion leaves;
- 50g cheese;
- 1 tbsp olive oil;
- Sea salt;
- Freshly ground pepper;

Process:
- Preheat the oven.
- Boil the potatoes and cut into slices.
- Place the tomato into hot water for 5 seconds, then into the ice one. Peel and cut into slices.
- Fry the potatoes with olive oil. Add tomato slices.
- Beat the eggs with salt and pepper, add the mixture to the potato and cook for 3-5 minutes.
- Sprinkle the omelet with grated cheese, place into the oven for 5 minutes and add some chopped onion leaves.

Spaghetti with fish, raisins and pine nuts

Ingredients:
- 200g spaghetti;
- 2 whitefish fillets;
- 2 tbsps raisins;
- 50g pine nuts;
- 1 fennel;
- 1 dry chili pepper;
- 1 tbsp rusks;
- Olive oil;
- Sea salt;
- Freshly ground pepper;

Process:
- Sprinkle whitefish fillets with salt and pepper, fry in a pan with olive oil until golden crust. The tear into pieces and make sure there are no any bones.
- Boil the spaghetti.
- Soak the raisins, fry the pine nuts.
- Cut the fennel.
- Heat the 1 tbsp olive oil in a deep pan, add chili pepper; fennel, raisins, half on the nuts, fish, add some water and cook for 1-2 minutes stirring occasionally.
- Add the sauce, the rest of the nuts and fennel to spaghetti. Sprinkle with rusks and olive oil.

Fish sticks

Ingredients:
- 450g salmon fillets;
- 650g potato;
- 200g frozen green peas;
- 1 egg;
- 3 tbsps flour;

- 2tsps lemon zest;
- 2 tbsps milk;
- 1 tbsp butter;
- Homemade breadcrumbs;
- Sea salt;
- Freshly ground pepper;

Process:
- Cut the fillet into slices (10cm long and 2-3cm wide).
- Combine flour, salt and pepper. Beat the egg. Add lemon zest to the breadcrumbs.
- Roll every slice of fish in flour, egg and breadcrumbs. Place in the fridge for 15 minutes.
- Peel the potato, cut into cubes and boil for 15 minutes. 2 minutes before cooked add green peas.
Then drain the water, add milk, butter and make puree.
- Place the fish sticks into the pan and fry for 10 minutes.
- Serve with puree.

Chicken rolls

Ingredients:
- 4 chicken breasts (skinless and boneless);
- 4 thin slices of cheese;
- 4 slices of ham;
- 150ml vegetable soup;
- 1 glove garlic;
- 1 laurel leaf;
- Chive leaves;
- ½ tsp cornstarch;
- 2 tbps sour cream;
- 1 tbsp salad oil;
- Sea salt;
- Freshly ground pepper;

Process:

- Preheat the oven to 350F.
- Cut the chicken breast into halves. Tenderize them. On each half put the slice of cheese and ham. Sprinkle it with salt and pepper, roll and fix with toothpicks.
- Cook the rolls in for 5 minutes until golden crust. Add garlic, laurel leaf, vegetable soup, cover and place them into the oven for 15-20 minutes.
- Cooked rolls put on a plate and cover with foil
- Take the soup from the rolls, boil it for 5 minutes. Add sour cream and cornstarch to the soup and boil for 1 minute stirring continuously until thick.
- Cut the rolls and serve with the sauce, herbs and vegetables.

Veal with sweet potato

Ingredients:
- 200g veal;
- 400g sweet potato;
- 300ml vegetable soup;
- 1 leek;
- 20g butter;
- 2 tbsps flour;
- 150ml orange juice;

Process:
- Preheat the oven to 360F.
- Wash and slice the leek.
- Stew the leek in a heat resistant pan.
- Cut the veal into cubes. Roll in the flour, place into the pan.
- Peel and chop the sweet potato and place into the pan.
- Add the juice and soup to the vegetables and meat. Bring to a boil, cover and place into the preheated oven for 75 minutes until tender.

Rabbit with crostini

Ingredients:
- Rabbit;
- Bread
- 4 cloves garlic;
- 2 leaves of rosemary;
- 8 leaves of sage;
- 8 leaves of parsley;
- 1 dry pepper;
- 2 tbsps white wine vinegar;
- Olive oil;
- ½ tsp sea salt;

Process:
- Skin, gut and cut the rabbit.
- Grind the garlic, rosemary, 3-4 sage leaves, and parsley in the mortar. Add 4 tbsps of olive oil, vinegar, salt and pepper.
- Heat the 2-3 tbsps of olive oil in a pan; cook the meat adding the mixture of herbs.
- Cook under the cover for 1 hour. Sprinkle with olive oil and the rest of the sage.
- Serve with toasted bread (crostini) or vegetables.

Small cutlets

Ingredients:
- 250g veal;
- 200g lean (chicken or pork)
- 1 tbsp tomato paste;
- Herbs;
- 1 tbsp flour;
- 2 tbsps sesame seeds;
- 1 tbsp salad oil

For sauce:
- 400g tomatoes;
- 1 clove garlic;
- 1 carrot;
- ½ tsp sugar;
- 1 tbsp olive oil;
- Sea salt;
- Freshly ground pepper;

Process:
- Preheat the oven for 350F.
- Put the meat through the meat-grinder, add tomato paste and herbs, mix well and make small patties. Roll in the flour, then in sesame seeds and place into the fridge.
- Place the tomatoes into hot water for 5 seconds, then into the ice one. Peel and cut into cubes. Grated carrot and minced garlic combine with salt.
- Mix olive oil, vegetables and sugar, place into pan and cook for 15 minutes. Also you can blend the sauce in a blender.
- Cook the patties with salad oil, dry them with paper towel, and then place into the oven for 5-10 minutes.
- Serve with the sauce.

Kebab on sticks

It is perfect for children's birthdays. Children like that meatballs look like an ice cream so they eat them with pleasure.

Ingredients:
- 450g lamb (no fat);
- 350g rice;
- 900ml vegetable soup;
- 175g frozen green peas;
- 1 onion;
- 1 shallot;

- ½ tsp paprika;
- ¼ tsp cinnamon;
- 1 leaf laurel;
- 2 cloves;
- ¼ tsp curcuma;
- 1 tbsp olive oil;
- Sea salt;
- Freshly ground pepper;

Process:
- Combine grated onion, salt, pepper, paprika, cinnamon and the grated lamb. Mix well and sprinkle with flour. Fire up the grill or preheat the oven with grill.
- Make patties. Put them on the sticks and grill for 20 minutes from both sides.
- Cook chopped shallot in the olive oi in a big pan. Place the rice into it, let it soak in the oil. Then add laurel leaf, curcuma, and cloves, pour vegetable soup, bring to a boil and cook for 10-15 minutes until the rice is tender. Two minutes before done add frozen peas.
- Serve with rice.

PASTRY AND DESSERTS

Pancakes for breakfast

Ingredients:
- 125g flour;
- ½ tsp leaven;
- 1 tbsp sugar;
- 1 egg;
- 150g butter milk;
- Sour cream;
- Fat;
- Pinch sea salt;

Process:
- Combine flour, leaven and salt in a bowl.
- Whip the egg with sugar, add butter milk. Mix it with previous mixture (flour, leaven and salt).
- Add 1 tbsp of salad oil and mix again.
- Heat a pan, add salad butter and bake small pancakes.
- Serve pancakes with sour cream.

Apricot puree

Ingredients:
- 225g dried apricots
- 450ml water;
- 2 tsps vanilla sugar or a few drops of vanilla extract;

Process:
- Place the dried apricots into the pot add some water to cover the fruits, bring to a boil, cover and boil over low heat for 25-30 minutes. Cook stirring and adding some water occasionally until tender.
- Turn off the gas and do not cover for 10 minutes to keep the flavor.
- Dilute vanilla sugar in boiled water and add the mixture to the puree. Then blend in a blender. If the mixture is too thick, add more water.

- Put the mixture into a bowl, wait until cool, cover and place into fridge.
- Instead of water you can use fresh orange juice so there would be no need in vanilla.

Muesli cookies

Ingredients:
- 125g sugar free muesli;
- 125 butter;
- 5 tbsps sugar;
- 1 egg;
- 50g coarse flour;
- 1 tsp leaven or ½ tsp baking powder;
- ½ tsp cinnamon;
- Sugar powder or dark chocolate;

Process:
- Preheat the oven to 370F.
- Combine sugar and butter and mix well.
- Add egg, muesli and mix well again.
- Add flour, leaven, cinnamon, pinch of salt and mix well.
- Make the balls size of walnut and put them on a baking pan.
- Press the balls down slightly with the help of the fork. Cook in the oven for 15 minutes until golden brown.
- Let them cool and then sprinkle with sugar powder. Or you can melt the chocolate and dip the cookies in it.

Carrot halva

Ingredients:
- 400g carrot;
- 300g sugar;
- 100g grated coconut;
- 75g raisin;

- 75g cashew;
- 1 tbsp butter;
- Pinch sea salt;

Process:
- Soak the raisins in 2 tbsps of boiled water.
- Grate the carrot finely.
- Heat the pan, add some butter and fry the cashew. Then pat them dry with paper towel.
- Mince the cashew.
- Pat the pan dry with paper towel. Add grated carrot and coconut and cook for 5-10 minutes stirring occasionally.
- Add sugar, salt and cook for another 10 minutes stirring continuously. Add the cashew and raisins, stir well and get off the flame.
- Line the bottom of a baking dish with a baking sheet. Cover the inside of buttered baking dish with the mixture. Leave for couple of hours and then cut into cubes.

Cream cheese bread

Ingredients:
- 2 cups wheat flour;
- 3 tbsps wheat germ;
- 100g cottage cheese;
- 100g grated cheese;
- 1 egg;
- 1 white of the egg;
- ½ cup rolled oats;
- ½ cup dates (or any other dried fruits)
- 1 tbsp flax seed;
- 1 tsp sesame seed;
- ½ tbsp yeast-powder;
- ¼ cup pineapple or apple juice;
- ½ cup water;

- 1 tbsp salad oil;
- ½ tsp sea salt;

Process:
- Preheat the oven to 370F.
- Blend wheat germs in a blender.
- Combine yeast-powder, flour, germs and salt in a bowl and mix well.
- Mix water and juice in a pot, add butter grated cottage cheese and cook over low heat stirring occasionally until smooth. Let it cool and then add the puree to the flour and yeast-powder. Add the egg and the white of it and mix well.
- Add rolled oats, mix well again, put the dough on a cutting board sprinkled with flour. Knead the dough until smooth and stick to hands. Make a ball, place it on the buttered baking dish. Cover with food wrap and put in a warm place.
- Remove pits from dates and cut the dates well.
- After proofing knead the dough thoroughly, add cheese, dates and place the dough into prepared pan. Sprinkle with flax and sesame seeds and place in the warm place for 10-15 minutes. Then place the dough into preheated oven and cook until golden brown.

Curd rice pudding

Ingredients:
- 400g curd;
- 200g rice;
- 600ml milk;
- 300g berries or dried fruits;
- 50g butter;
- 150g sugar;
- A few drops of vanilla extract;
- Sugar powder;

Process:
- Preheat the oven to 340F.
- Pour the milk in a pot and bring it to a boil.

- Add rice, cover and boil over low heat until cooked. Then let it cool.
- Separate the white from the yolk.
- Combine the yolks with melted butter, sugar and curd.
- Beat the egg whites until stiff and add it to the curd.
- Add vanilla extract and berries to the rice and mix well.
- Combine the rice and curd, mix well and put it into the buttered baking dish. Place into the oven and bake for 30-35 minutes.
- Sprinkle cooked pudding with sugar powder.

Apple pie with raisin and hazelnut

Ingredients:
- 450g apples;
- 120g raisin;
- 350g flour;
- 170g sugar;
- 2 eggs;
- 20g hazelnut;
- Juice and zest of 1 lemon;
- 1 tsp yeast powder;
- 1 tbsp wine vinegar;
- 150ml salad butter;
- Sea salt;

Process:
- Preheat the oven to 360F.
- Soak the raisins in the warm water for 10 minutes and then drain the water.
- Remove the seeds and cut the apples into cubes. Sprinkle them with lemon juice to prevent потемнеть.
- Cut the lemon zest into thin strips.
- Place the olive oil, sugar and eggs in food processor and process until smooth.
- Continue stirring and add flour, salt and yeast powder.

- Add apples, raisins and lemon zest to the dough. Mix well.
- Place the dough on the buttered baking dish. Sprinkle with hazelnuts.
- Cover the pie with baking sheet and bake for 30 minutes. Then remove the sheet and bake for another 30 minutes.

Curd roulade with candied fruits

Ingredients:
- 500g cottage cheese;
- 100g butter;
- Handful of candied fruits;
- 4 eggs;
- 2 cups sugar;
- 2 tbsps flour;
- 2 tbsps corn starch;

Process:
- Preheat the oven to 360F.
- Separate the white from the yolk.
- Whip 4 yolks with a cup of sugar.
- Beat the egg whites until stiff and combine with yolks.
- Add flour stirring continuously (remove any lumps).
- Pour the batter on the buttered baking dish and bake in the oven for 20 minutes.
- Strain the curd through the sieve, add the rest of the sugar, corn starch and melted butter. Mix everything well.
- Add candied fruits and mix well.
- When done, take it out of the oven, cover with mixture of fried fruits and curd on it and roll it up.

School

School is a big challenge both for children and parents. It is like the end of unclouded childhood and the start of real adult life.

And because of these hints of adult life sometime children get rebellious. Once my children organized a delegation and demanded for a day off. I agreed, but asked to make a schedule for me – so that I could know how they were going to spend their life. After a quick consultation they gave me a paper:

8.10 – breakfast (10 minutes later than usual)

After that – games.

9.30 – swimming pool, though we never go to the swimming pool so early – the water is too cold. I tried to bring it to their notice but was ignored.

13.40 – dinner. Usually at 10am they eat fruits or drink juice to maintain the energy. But they skip it. I told them that they would starve to death but was ignored. Again.

Then there was a nap (with their politburo decision they reduced it to one hour and demanded to wake them up). Then there was lunch, riding a bike and finally a sapper in 18.55 (usually at 19.00). I couldn't help but ask:

- Why not 18.52?

But they were not confused and insisted on this time. I took a red pen and wrote "APPROVED". And then I told my children:

- Well, we signed this agreement. In conclusion you didn't mention juice or fruits before dinner so you will not get them. Moreover, there were no sweets, no trips in you agreement so you can't demand it from me.

And now they were confused. They asked to make a new agreement but I said it was too late.

It was a great experience to see how unique your children are, how they protect their views.

AFTER 7 YEARS BREAKFAST

Granola – homemade muesli

Ingredients:
- 300g oatmeal;
- 200g almonds;
- 100g sunflower seeds (peeled)
- 80g sesame seeds;
- 50g brown sugar;
- 6 tbsps liquid honey;
- 250g raisins;
- 2 tsps cinnamon;
- 1 tsps dry ginger;
- 2 tbsps salad oil;
- 1 tbsp butter;
- 1 tsp salt;

Process:
- Preheat the oven to 340F.
- Combine oatmeal, almonds, sunflower seeds, sesame seeds, sugar, cinnamon and ginger. Add honey and raisins and mix well.
- Place on a baking dish covered with buttered baking sheet. Cook for 40 minutes stirring occasionally. Sprinkle with salt and let it cool.

Omelette roll-ups

Ingredients:
- 4 eggs;
- 4 sun-dried tomatoes;
- Lavash;
- Herbs;

- Olive oil;
- Sea salt;

Process:
- Beat the eggs. Slice the tomatoes and add them to the eggs. Add some salt.
- Heat some olive oil in a pan and cook the egg mixture until cooked.
- Cut the omelette into halves. Put them on the lavash, sprinkle with herbs and roll it up.

Fresh tomato sauce

Ingredients:
- 2 tomatoes;
- 1 leaf scallion (chopped);
- Handful of cilantro or parsley (finely chopped);
- 1 tsp lemon juice;
- ¼ tsp sugar;
- Sea salt;
- Freshly ground pepper;

Process:
- Blanch tomatoes in boiling water for a minute. Then remove and transfer to a bowl of cold water. When cold enough to handle, gently remove the skin and cut into small cubes.
- Combine all the ingredients, add lemon juice, sugar, salt and pepper to taste.

Omlette with secret

Ingredients:
- 3 eggs;
- fat;
- Sea salt;
- Freshly ground pepper;

Beat the eggs, add salt and pepper to taste. Heat some fat in a pan, then cover the bottom of the pan with beaten eggs (like a thin pancake). Place the filling on the one side of the omelette and cover with another side.

Filling with tomatoes

Ingredients:
- 1 tomato;
- Leaves of scallion;

Remove the skin of tomato. Cut all the ingredients and stew them.

Filling with chicken and cucumber

Ingredients:
- 1 boiled chicken breast;
- 1 cucumber;
- Herbs;
- Sea salt;
- Freshly ground pepper;

Cut all the ingredients into small cubes. Add salt and pepper to taste and mix well.

Secret tomato sauce

Ingredients:
- 400g tomatoes;
- ½ carrot;
- ½ zucchini;
- 1 onion;
- ½ leek (only white part);
- 2 garlic cloves;
- ½ sweet red pepper;
- 150ml vegetable soup;
- 1 tbsp olive oil;
- 1 tbsp tomato paste;
- ½ sugar;
- Herbs;
- Sea salt;

- Freshly ground pepper;

Process:
- Grate the carrot and zucchini. Cut onion, leek and garlic finely, but don't mix.
- Blanch tomatoes in boiling water for a minute. Then remove and transfer to a bowl of cold water. When cold enough to handle, gently remove the skin and cut into small cubes.
- Roast the pepper in the oven, remove the skin and cut into cubes.
- Heat the olive oil in a pan, add onion and leek and cook until soft.
- Add garlic. A few minutes later add pepper, tomatoes, tomato paste, sugar, carrot and zucchini. Cook for 5 minutes stirring occasionally.
- Add the vegetable soup, salt and pepper to taste and cook over low heat for 25-30 minutes stirring continuously.
- At the end of cooking add chopped herbs.

Lavash and sweet pepper

Ingredients:
- 1 red sweet pepper;
- 1 yellow sweet pepper;
- 1 red onion;
- 2 garlic cloves;
- Lavash;
- Cheese;
- Fat;
- Sour cream;
- Olive oil;
- Sea salt;
- Freshly ground pepper;

Process:
- Preheat the oven to 360F.
- Remove peduncles and seeds of pepper and cut into thin strips.
- Peel the onion and garlic. Cut the onion into rounds, and chop the garlic.

- Heat some olive oil in a pan, and stew the vegetables until tender. Add salt and pepper to taste.
- Heat the lavash or pita in the oven. Place the steamed veggies on it, sprinkle with grated cheese, and put some sour cream on top. You can roll it up or cover with another pita. Place into the oven for 3-5 minutes.

Guacamole for children

Ingredients:
- 1 avocado;
- ½ sweet pepper;
- 1 tsp curd for infants;
- ½ tsp lemon juice;
- Sea salt;

Process:
- Peel the avocado, remove the pit and blend until smooth.
- Cut the pepper and combine with avocado puree.
- Add curd, salt and mi well.

Sweet bar "Health"

Ingredients:
- 250g oatmeal;
- 125g dried apricot;
- 75g raisins;
- 75g almond;
- 50g sesame seeds;
- 150g butter;
- 150g sugar;
- 100g liquid honey;

Process:
- Preheat the oven to 380F.
- Cover the bottom of baking dish with buttered baking sheet.

- Combine minced almond, chopped dried apricot, sesame seeds and oatmeal.
- Melt the butter, add sugar and honey and cook on a low heat until completely dissolved.
- After that mix butter mixture with the rest of the ingredients, put in the baking dish and cook in the oven for 15-20 minutes until golden brown.
- Take it out of the oven, let it cool and place into the fridge for 1-2 hours. Then cut it into thick stripes.

Meat casserole

Ingredients:
- 250g beef mince;
- 250g pork mince;
- 2 loaves of white bread;
- 2 tbsps milk;
- 1 egg;
- 1 onion;
- 2 garlic cloves;
- 1 tsp herbs;
- 1 tsp tomato paste;
- Sea salt;
- Freshly ground pepper;

For tomato sauce:
- 400 tomatoes;
- 1 onion;
- 1 garlic clove;
- Parsley;
- 1 tbsp salad oil;

Process:
- Preheat the oven to 380F.
- Whip the egg with milk. Cut the bread into small pieces and soak them in the milk with egg. Left for 5 minutes.

- Combine both minces, chopped garlic, onion, herbs and tomato paste. Mix well. Add soaked bread, salt and pepper and mix again. Place the meat mixture in buttered roasting dish and cook in the oven for 50 minutes.
- To make the sauce heat the oil in a pan. Add chopped onion, garlic and cook until tender. Add tomatoes and cook over low heat for 15 minutes.
- Serve the casserole with tomato sauce.

Homemade hamburger with chicken cutlet

Ingredients:
- 350g chicken mince;
- 50g brisket or bacon;
- 50g oatmeal;
- 1 egg;
- ½ tsp herbs de Provence;
- Pita;
- 2 cucumbers;
- 2 tomatoes;
- Salad leaves;
- Sea salt;
- Freshly ground pepper;

Process:
- Chicken mince combine with chopped brisket, oatmeal, beaten egg, herbs, salt and pepper. With wet hands make 8-10 patties. They should be about 2cm thick.
- Heat a grill pan.
- Grease the patties with some oil, place them on a dry grill pan. Cook for 5 minutes in each side. Repeat (each side of a cutlet should be cooked twice).
- Wash the cucumbers and tomatoes, cut them into rounds. Tear the leaves of salad with your hands.
- Cut the pita into halves. Place on one half cucumber, tomatoes, salad leaves and then cutlet. Cover it with another half.

Banana cupcake

Ingredients:

- 125g flour;
- 125g crude flour;
- 125g sugar;
- 2 bananas;
- 150ml salad oil;
- Grated zest and juice of ½ orange;
- 2tsps leaven;
- 1tsp cinnamon;
- 75g walnut;
- Sea salt;

Process:

- Preheat the oven to 360F.
- Combine flour, cinnamon, leaven and minced nuts in a bowl.
- Combine sugar, pinch of salt and oil in another bowl. Mix well.
- Beat eggs, blended bananas, zest and juice.
- Combine two mixtures.
- Place the batter in a baking dish covered with buttered baking sheet and bake in the preheated oven for 50 minutes.
- Take the cake out of the oven, let it cool.

HOT MEAL

Spaghetti with chicken liver

Ingredients:
- 250g chicken liver;
- 100g spaghetti;
- 60g bacon;
- 4 garlic cloves;
- 2 chili pepper;
- Parsley;
- 3 tbsps flour;
- 3 tbsps vegetable soup;
- 3 tbsps olive oil;
- Sea salt;
- Freshly ground pepper;

Process:
- Fry the chopped bacon in a pan.
- Combine flour, salt and pepper in a bowl. Roll the liver in this mixture and cook it with bacon for 2-3 minutes.
- Pour the vegetable soup and cook for another 2-3 minutes.
- To make the sauce heat the olive oil in a pan, and add chopped garlic, chopped parsley and chili pepper.
- Boiled spaghetti dress with the sauce and add liver with bacon.

Spaghetti with sweet pepper

Ingredients:
- 300g spaghetti;
- 2 sweet red peppers;
- Handful of almonds;
- Parsley;

- 50g grated cheese;
- 40ml olive oil;
- Sea salt;
- Freshly ground pepper;

Process:
- Preheat the oven to 360F.
- Place the peppers on a roasting dish and place them in the oven for 20 minutes. Then let them cool for 5 minutes and remove the skin and seeds.
- Blend almonds, peppers, parsley and olive oil. Add salt and pepper to taste, grated cheese, 2tbsps water and blend until smooth.
- Dress the boiled spaghetti with the sauce. Serve hot.

Potato with filling

Ingredients:
- 2 big potatoes;
- brisket;
- 2 tbsps milk;
- 30g fat;
- 150g cheese;
- Scallion;
- Sea salt;

Process:
- Preheat the oven to 360F.
- Wash the potatoes, jab with toothpick or fork. And bake in the oven for 45 minutes until tender.
- Take cooked potatoes out of the oven and let them cool.
- Melt the fat in the oven, and add the brisket cut into cubes, cook over the low heat and place on a plate.
- Place the chopped scallion in the pan and cook for 2-3 minutes.
- Cut the potatoes into halves, remove the core and blend it with milk until smooth. Add the brisket, scallion and half of the grated cheese to the puree. Add salt to taste.

- Place the puree in the center of potato, sprinkle with the rest of the grated cheese. Cover with foil and place in the oven for 10 minutes.

Potato pie with meat

Ingredients:
- 200g chicken;
- 200g turkey;
- 700g potato;
- 400g tomatoes;
- 250ml vegetable soup;
- 1 carrot;
- 1 onion;
- 1 celeriac;
- 3 garlic cloves;
- 2 tbsps lentils;
- 1 tsp herbs;
- 125g frozen green pea;
- 50g cheese;
- 2 tbsps milk;
- Salad oil';
- Sea salt;
- Freshly ground pepper;

Process:
- Preheat the oven to 400F.
- Put meat through a meat-grinder. Chop the onion and garlic and cut the celeriac into rounds.
- Place the minced meat in a pan and cook until done. Add the lentils, peas, tomatoes, vegetable soup, herbs, salt and pepper, bring to a boil and simmer for 40 minutes.
- Peel the carrot and potatoes, cut into cubes and boil for 15 minutes until done. Drain the water. Pour hot milk, add salt and pepper and make a puree.

- Put the minced meat into a baking dish, cover with the puree and place into the oven for 15-20 minutes until the top is golden brown. Sprinkle with cheese.

Meat and vegetables in a wok

Ingredients:
- 300g filets of beef;
- 150g green beans;
- 150g frozen green peas;
- 1 pack of rice noodles;
- Water or vegetable soup;
- 1 ginger root;
- 2 carrots;
- 4 leaves of scallion;
- 2 tsps gingili oil;
- 2 tbsps soy sauce;
- 1 tbsp cider vinegar;
- 1 tbsp salad oil;
- ½ tsp starch;

Process:
- Cut the meat into stripes, remove the fat, put in a bowl, and add 1 tsp gingili oil, soy sauce and cider vinegar.
- Add grated ginger with its juice to the meat and leave for 10 minutes.
- Cut the carrots into stripes.
- Bring water or vegetable soup to a boil, add spaghetti and cook for 10 minutes.
- Heat a wok, add gingili and salad oil and cook meat for 2 minutes until golden brown.
- Remove the meat with a skimmer, put the carrot in the wok, and then add green beans, frozen peas and chopped scallion and cook for 3-5 minutes.
- Combine starch and marinade, pour 5 tbsps of vegetable soup and put everything in the wok. Add meat and spaghetti, cook for 1 minute and serve.

Sole with grapes

Ingredients:
- 8 sole fillets;
- 1 tbsp flour;
- 20g butter;
- 75g mushrooms;
- 100ml vegetable soup;
- 100ml rich cream;
- 1 tsp lemon juice;
- 2 tbsps chopped parsley;
- 20 berries of sultana (white grape without seeds);
- Sea salt;
- Freshly ground pepper;

Process:
- Roll the fish in flour and seasonings. Melt the half of the butter in a big pan and fry the fish over medium heat for 2 minutes from both sides until golden brown. Put it on a plate and let it cool.
- Cut the mushrooms, melt the rest of the butter in the pan and cook mushrooms for 3 minutes.
- Pour the vegetable soup and stew over a low heat for 2 minutes.
- Mix with cream and lemon juice and stew for another 2 minutes.
- Add parsley, grapes cut into halves, salt and pepper. Cover the fish with this sauce.

Fish rissoles

Ingredients:
- 180g tuna;
- 600g potato;
- 1 tbsp butter;
- 2 tbsps chopped parsley;
- 200g corn;
- 2 tbsps flour;
- 1 salad oil;

- Sea salt;
- Freshly ground pepper;

Process:
- Boil the potatoes.
- Drain the water, add the butter to the potatoes and make a puree.
- Add the chopped parsley, salt and pepper to the puree.
- Add tuna and corn and mix well.
- Make the patties and roll them in flour.
- Heat the oil in a pan and fry the patties for 3-4 minutes from both sides until golden brown.

Place them on a paper towel.
- Serve with salad or vegetables.

Fish casserole

Ingredients:
- 450g lancet fish;
- 125g frozen shrimps;
- 450g potato;
- 225g batata;
- 1 zucchini;
- 450ml milk;
- 150ml vegetable soup;
- 3 tbsps butter;
- 50g flour;
- 1 tbsp lemon juice;
- 2 tbsps chopped parsley;
- Sea salt;
- Freshly ground pepper;

Process:
- Heat 2 tbsps of butter in a pan, add flour, and pour the soup, milk and lemon juice.
- Bring to a boil and cook for 1-2 minutes until thick.

- Get the pan off the flame and add the chopped fish and shrimps to the sauce.
- Peel the potatoes and boil them with zucchini for 10 minutes until tender.
- Grate the potatoes, batata and zucchini and combine everything together and mix well. Put it on the fish.
- Melt the rest of the butter and pour it on the casserole. Add salt and pepper and place into the oven for 25 minutes until golden brown.
- Sprinkle with chopped parsley.

Turkey cutlets with beans

Ingredients:
- 500-600g minced turkey;
- 150-200g green bean;
- 300ml water;
- 1 leek (only white part);
- 2-5 garlic cloves;
- 5 tbsps olive oil;
- 1 tsp butter;
- 2 tsps balsamic reduction;
- 1 bay leaf;
- Finely grated zest of 1 orange;
- ¼ tsp nutmeg;
- 1 tsp herbs;
- 1 tsp peppercorns;
- 1 tsp sea salt;

Process:
- Preheat the oven to 360F.
- Soak the beans for 4 hours and then boil them.
- Mince pepper and salt. Peel the garlic and cut it.
- Add herbs, half of the pepper with salt, 2 tbsps of olive oil, 2 tsps of balsamic reduction, zest, nutmeg, garlic, bay leaf to the minced turkey and mix well.

- Place the mixture in a bowl and cover it with food wrap, place it in the fridge for a night. Remove the bay leaf, mix well again and make patties.
- Heat 2 tbsps of olive oil in a pan. Fry the patties from both sides until golden brown. Add beans and sprinkle with salt and pepper.
- Heat 1 tbsp of butter and olive oil in a pot, add leek cut into rounds, garlic, 1 tsp balsamic reduction and 300ml of water. Bring to a boil.
- Pour the cutlets with the sauce and place into the preheated oven for 30 minutes.

Spicy chicken

Ingredients:
- 1 chicken carcass;
- 300ml thick yoghurt;
- 150ml coconut milk;
- 100ml vegetable soup;
- 1 onion;
- 2 garlic cloves;
- 1 tsp coriander seeds;
- 1 tsp caraway;
- 1 tsp cumin;
- ½ tsp corn;
- ½ tsp ginger;
- ½ tsp corn flour;
- Handful of fresh cilantro;
- 1 tbsp of salad oil;

Process:
- Separate the chicken meat from the bones, and cut it into big cubes.
- Peel the garlic and onion and cut.
- Heat the salad oil in a pan. Add the onion and garlic, cook well, and then add other seasonings.
- Combine corn flour and yogurt, pour in the pan. Then pour vegetable soup and coconut milk.
- Put the chicken in the pan, cover and cook over a medium heat for 20 minutes.

- Sprinkle the chicken with cilantro. Serve with rice or vegetable salad.

Chicken with mushrooms

Ingredients:
- 3 chicken breasts (skinless and boneless);
- 125g mushrooms;
- 600ml milk;
- 40g flour;
- Pinch of herbs;
- Phyllo dough;
- 1 tbsp salad oil;
- Fat;
- Sea salt;
- Freshly ground pepper;

Process:
- Preheat the oven to 380F.
- Heat the fat in a pan, add mushrooms and cook for 5-6 minutes. Then add salt and pepper to taste. Remove the mushrooms with skimmer.
- Combine flour and milk and pour the mixture in the pan. Add herbs and cook over a medium heat stirring continuously until thick.
- Cut the chicken breasts into cubes, mix them with sauce and stew over a low heat for 3-4 minutes. Then add salt and pepper, mushrooms and put in a roasting dish.
- Cut the dough into pieces. Each buttered piece put on the chicken.
- Place into the oven and cook for 25 minutes until golden brown.

PASTRY, DESSERTS

Curd rosettes

Ingredients:
- 250g curd;
- 100g butter;
- 450g flour;
- 2 yolks;
- ½ cup sugar;
- 1/3 tsp yeast-powder;
- 1 tsp lemon juice;
- 1 tsp vanilla sugar;

Process:
- Preheat the oven to 340F.
- Combine butter, curd, sugar and yolks. Add yeast-powder, vanilla sugar, flour and mix well. Split into 4 parts.
- Roll out one part of the dough and with the help of the mug or cup make rounds.
- Roll up on of the rounds, another wrap round it. Then add 2-3 rounds more to make a rose.
- Make the bottom flat.
- Place the rosettes on a baking dish and cook in the oven for 15 minutes until golden brown.

Muffins with blueberry

Ingredients:
- 225g flour;
- 300ml milk;
- 150 fresh blueberry (or any other frozen berries);
- 100g sugar;
- 50g oatmeal;
- 1 egg;
- 1 pack of leaven;

- 6 tbsps salad oil;
- Some drops of vanilla extract;
- Sugar powder;
- Sea salt;

Process:
- Preheat the oven to 380F.
- Combine flour, leaven, sugar and pinch of salt in a bowl.
- In another bowl combine egg, milk, butter, blueberry and vanilla extract. Then add oatmeal and mix everything well.
- Leave the mixture for 10 minutes.
- Add the mixture from the first bowl to the oatmeal and mix well.
- Pour the batter in buttered cake pans and place into the preheated oven. Bake for 20 minutes until golden brown.
- Let the muffin cool for 10 minutes and sprinkle them with sugar powder.

Curd croissants

Ingredients:
- 250g curd;
- 200g butter;
- 2 cups flour;
- 1 yolk;
- 1 tbsp milk;
- Sesame seeds;
- Poppy seeds;
- Jam;

Process:
- Preheat the oven to 400F.
- Combine curd, flour, melted butter, mix everything well and split into two parts.
- Roll out the half, cut it into triangles and roll into croissants. Put into each croissant ½ tsp of jam.
- Roll out another part of the dough. Then cut into stripes, fold in half and convolve.

- Whip the yolk with milk and coat each croissant. Then sprinkle them with sesame and poppy seeds.
- Bake in the oven until golden brown.

Chocolate cheesecake

Ingredients:
- 500g farmer cheese;
- 120g flour;
- 110g butter;
- 5 eggs;
- 1 chocolate bar;
- 60g raisin;
- 3 tbsps potato starch;
- 90g sugar;
- Finely grated zest of 1 orange;
- 2 tbsps cold water;
- 2 tbsps hot water;
- Sea salt;

Process:
- Preheat the oven to 380F.
- Put flour through a sieve and add a pinch of salt.
- Cut 60g of cooled butter into cubes. Combine the butter with flour, and pour cold water. Very quickly roll up the dough, wrap in plastic and place into the fridge.
- Place the raisin into a small pot, add 2 tbsps of hot water and cook over a low heat for 5 minutes.
- Separate 4 yolks from the whites.
- Combine curd and sugar, and add 1 egg and 4 yolks, raisins, orange zest and starch.
- Whip the whites with pinch of salt and add them to the mixture.
- Place the dough in the buttered baking dish, cover with baking sheet and place into the preheated oven for 5 minutes.
- Melt the chocolate and butter.

- Put the curd mixture on the dough, pour with melted chocolate and bake in the oven for 45-50 minutes.

Poppy rolled cake

Ingredients:
- 70g flour;
- 350ml milk;
- 80g sugar;
- 60g butter;
- 15g fresh yeast;
- 1 egg;
- 1 yolk;
- Sugar powder;

For filling:
- 250g poppy seeds;
- 100g sugar;
- 150g almonds;
- 60g butter;
- Zest of 3 lemons;
- 4 tsps honey;

Process:
- Preheat the oven to 360F.
- Pour 300ml of milk in a pot and bring it to a boil. Then add butter and 65g of sugar. Mix everything well and let it cool.
- The rest of the milk (it should be warm) combine with yeast, egg, the rest of the sugar and 1 tbsp of flour. Mix everything well and put into a warm place for 10-15 minutes.
- Mix both milk mixtures, add the rest of the flour and stir until smooth. Put into a buttered bowl, cover with towel and put into the warm place for 1 hour.

- To make the feeling soak the poppy seeds with water (it should be fully covered), and cook over a low heat for 40 minutes. Drain the water, blend the sesame seeds until powder. Add sugar, minced almonds, butter, lemon zest and honey. Mix everything well.
- Split the dough into two parts and roll them out. Spread the filling and roll the dough up. Coat with beaten egg white and bake in the oven for 25 minutes. Sprinkle with sugar powder.

Carrot cake with almonds

Ingredients:
- 200g carrot;
- 200g sour cream;
- 100g almond;
- 1 ½ cup sugar;
- 1 cup flour;
- 3 eggs;
- ½ bar of white chocolate;
- 1 tsp vanilla sugar;
- ½ yeast-powder;
- 1 tsp lemon juice;
- Pinch of sea salt;

Process:
- Preheat the oven to 400F.
- Whip the eggs with 1 cup of sugar, add yeast-powder and lemon juice, salt, flour, grated carrot and mix everything well until thick (thicker than sour cream).
- Add minced almonds to the batter.
- Pour the batter in the buttered baking dish and bake in the oven for 20 minutes. Then reduce the heat to 300F and bake for another 15 minutes. Cool it and take out of the dish.
- Combine sour cream, sugar and vanilla sugar and whip until thick.
- Cut the pie shell into halves. Cover them with cream and combine again. Sprinkle the top with grated white sugar.

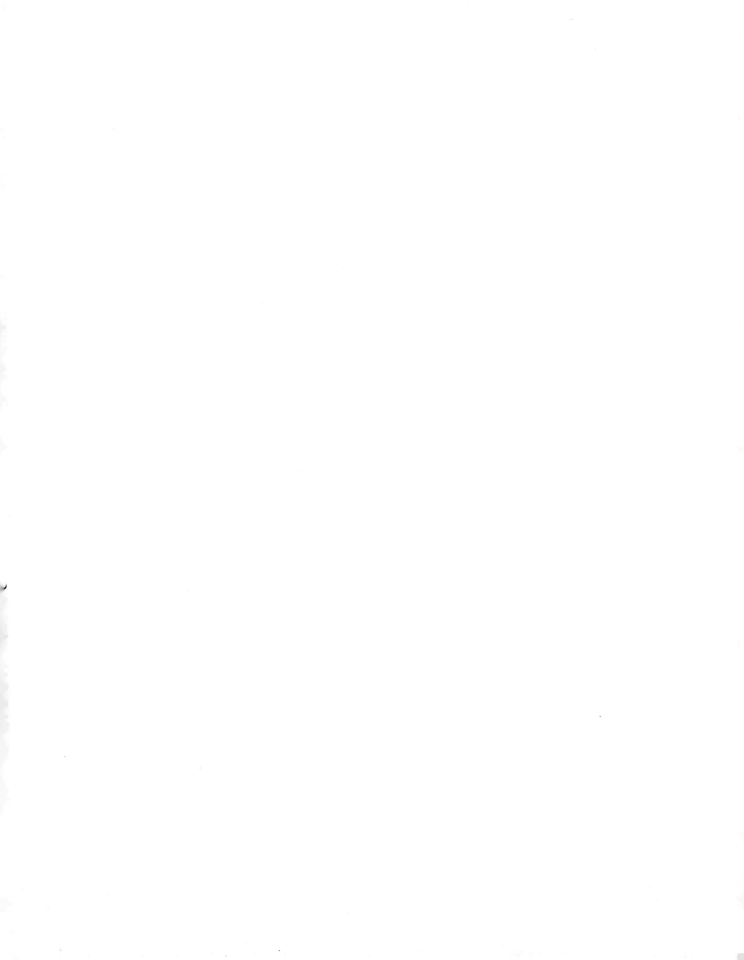

CPSIA information can be obtained
at www.ICGtesting.com
Printed in the USA
BVHW091029210721
612411BV00014B/4233